Advance Praise for
IT'S A SISTAH THING

"Monique Brown understands that Black women must be proactive about our health. When she discovered she had fibroid tumors, Monique researched, questioned, probed and devoured every bit of information she could find on the subject. Now sisters like me, who also suffer with fibroids, have this wonderful book, a one-stop source to aid in our healing."
—Monique Greenwood, author of *Having What Matters:*
The Black Women's Guide to Creating the Life You Really Want

"At last . . . a heartfelt and practical book that sheds light on a problem which has plagued so many of us for so long. Thanks for having our back. Monique . . . it truly is a Sistah thing!"
—Terrie M. Williams, author, founder of The Stay Strong Foundation

"Finally, a thorough guide for black women who have fibroids. In *It's a Sistah Thing,* Monique Brown brings together mounds of research, expert advice and real-women stories that will help sisters struggling with benign uterine tumors. This is an empowering text that requires us to take action and take responsibility for our health. It covers the very latest in medical and nonmedical solutions. It offers checklists and interactive exercises to help guide us through the maze of options. Perhaps most important, the book is funny, hopeful and inspirational. By sharing her own personal history with fibroids and compiling a wealth of fibroid facts, Monique Brown has written an indispensible guide for black women."
—Ziba Kashef, author of *Like a Natural Woman: The Black Woman's*
Guide to Alternative Healing and Disease Prevention

"Reading this book was like talking to a good friend. It is thoroughly researched and covers not only traditional approaches to the treatment of fibroids, but nontraditional methods as well. If you or someone you care about has fibroids, this book will be invaluable."
—Hilda Hutcherson, M.D., gynecologist, author of
What Your Mother Never Told You About Sex

"Monique Brown's groundbreaking book is packed with useful and important information that's designed to bring great comfort and relief. She has thoroughly researched and written it with great care that sisters may enjoy healthier and happier lives."
—Dr. Grace Cornish, author of *10 Good Choices*
That Empower Black Women's Lives

It's A
Sistah Thing

A Guide to Understanding and Dealing with Fibroids for Black Women

Monique R. Brown

Foreword by Ifeanyi C.O. Obiakor, M.D.

Illustrations by William Acvedo

KENSINGTON PUBLISHING CORP.
http://www.kensingtonbooks.com

This book presents information based upon the research and personal experiences of the author. It is not intended to be a substitute for a professional consultation with a physician or other health-care provider. Neither the publisher nor the author can be held responsible for any adverse effects or consequences resulting from the use of any of the information in this book. They also cannot be held responsible for any errors or omissions in the book. If you have a condition that requires medical advice, the publisher and the author urge you to consult a competent health-care professional.

DAFINA BOOKS are published by

Kensington Publishing Corp.
850 Third Avenue
New York, NY 10022

CONTENTS

FOREWORD

I initially met Monique Brown on May 2, 2000. The visit was memorable, to say the least. Apparently, I was among a long list of physicians that Monique saw regarding her fibroids and she was openly frustrated and upset. I listened to Monique's tearful rendition detailing her host of complaints regarding her condition, examined her, and offered the same conclusion that the many doctors before me had provided. Given the size of the fibroids, her symptoms, and her undying desire to have children, I believed that Monique would get relief only if the myomas were surgically removed by a myomectomy, a surgical procedure that I hoped would keep her uterus intact so she could eventually conceive.

I made no guarantees about the results, however. I told her up front that this type of surgery had possible complications, such as excessive bleeding that could result in the performance of an emergency hysterectomy. Even if the surgery was performed without a hitch, there was also the possibility that internal adhesions could develop from the surgery and this condition could also cause infertility. In addition, there was a chance that the fibroids could return after the myomectomy was performed and those myomas could also be problematic. The bottom line was that the best answer I could give Monique as to whether or not she'd ever be able to conceive was a definite "maybe."

Of course, that wasn't the response Monique wanted to hear. She came to my office in search of a miracle and I could only offer more of the mundane—the same facts that she had come across again and again. But what else could I do? Conventional medical options are limited when it comes to the treatment of fibroids.

Still, I somehow felt compelled to do more or at the very least say more. So I reached out and offered a hug. "We'll get through this," I said. "And you will smile again." She looked at me as if she wanted to believe me, but I didn't think that she did. Based on how that visit went, I concluded that I'd probably never see Monique Brown again. But I was wrong. That visit was the first of many sessions that followed. Eventually, Monique scheduled her myomectomy for Thursday, August 17. Although the visits leading up to the surgery were just as tearful, if not more so, than Monique's first visit, it seemed that she was attempting to take charge of her health—at least to some degree. Each time Monique came into the office, she had a heap of questions that she wanted answered and mounds of research that she wanted clarified. Some of it was overkill, but I think she gained confidence as she became more informed about her condition and the surgery. It seemed as if she was transforming from victim to victor.

If I'd had any doubts about Monique's desire to take an active role in her health, those doubts were put to rest on the day of the surgery. Prior to the eight A.M. operation, Monique quizzed me along with my team of surgical experts—the anesthesiologist, resident, and other attending physician—about various phases of the surgery. She took a close look at her chart and got a detailed explanation of the results and how those findings were going to impact her surgery. It was only after she was satisfied with the responses that Monique agreed to go forward with the procedure. I'm sure my colleagues were just as surprised as I was by the feisty patient. But despite the surprise, they also appreciated her candor and concern. That was demonstrated vividly when Monique was recovering because each one of the physicians that were in the operating room felt compelled to pay our most "inquisitive" patient a personal visit. And even though my partner, Barbara Gordon, did not participate in this particular surgery, she took it upon herself to personally see how Monique was doing. Apparently, if patients show a special interest in their health care, that enthusiasm rubs off on their physicians.

The surgery went well. And while I could tell that by looking at the chart, the grin across Monique's face was all the proof I needed. Even though Monique was still a little sore from the myomectomy, she was laughing and telling jokes. She greeted me with an excitement that I had never witnessed in my office, and just as I had promised months earlier, she was smiling again.

Now Monique smiles often and I'm not at all surprised by her list of questions during office visits. It's a part of the process. In fact, I find it makes my job easier when patients are well informed and are active participants in their health care.

For this reason, I think a book such as this is especially important. It's packed with just about everything you need to know about fibroids and offered in a friendly conversational style that's easy to understand. Once you complete these chapters and the accompanying interactive exercises, you'll be able to manage your fibroid condition and make decisions regarding your treatment. Plus, you'll have uncovered some techniques to improve communication between you and your physician.

Further, you'll discover how other black women, fibroids' biggest victims, handled their own conditions. These anecdotes are essential because they serve as proof that you are not alone in your quest for better fibroid care. A successful treatment plan requires a series of partnerships between you and your physician, you and other fibroid sufferers, as well as you and your loved ones. As long as you're willing to take the first step, you can use this book and your fibroids to help you bridge the gap and open up a world of possibilities in this area of medicine.

Ifeanyi C. O. Obiakor, M.D. F.A.C.O.G.
Obstetrician/gynecologist based in Brooklyn, New York

ACKNOWLEDGMENTS

Dear God, thanks so much for all of your blessings. They've been so plentiful I almost don't know where to begin. Somehow, some way, you always seem to put me in touch with the right people at the right time. And although I once thought that my string of misfortunes was the beginning of the end, I now realize that some things had to end so I could enjoy the fruits of a new beginning.

Dr. Obiakor, who would have thought that my first visit to your office would lead to all of this? Not only have you become my favorite doctor, you've also become my confidant and dear friend. Your participation exceeded my wildest expectations and dreams. Without the support of you and your partner, Dr. Barbara Gordon, this project would not have been possible. Thank you both for going above and beyond the call of duty—it was much appreciated.

Dad, you can exhale now. Your daughter is now an author, so you have officially earned your bragging rights. I couldn't have done any of this without the overwhelming support of you and Mom. Who else would have driven more than five hundred miles to give me their computer when mine took a dive? Only two loving parents like you—thank you, Herman and Margaret Brown.

I'd like to give a rousing round of applause for my agent Barbara Lowenstein and editor Karen Thomas at Kensington for believing in this project and seeing it through to the finish. I'd also like to praise my fabulous editorial duo—Leslie E. Royal and Tara Lawrence—for pulling together the research and editing at lightning speed with minutes to spare. You done good (I guess you missed this one).

Hey, William Acevedo, you were right. A Latino can do a great job illustrating a black book. You did your thing—gracias.

I'd also like to offer my appreciation to the kind hearts that allowed me to use their computers when I couldn't access mine or it was on the blink—Paula Pelliccia, Rodney and Stephanie Brown, and Derek T. Dingle. And I certainly can't forget to give a nod to everyone that helped me maneuver through the publishing process—Terrie Williams, Monique Greenwood, Carolyn Brown, Dr. Grace Cornish, Wendy Harris, Cheryl Wadlington, Linda Iloba, and everyone else who freely shared knowledge.

And many, many thanks to all of you sisterfriends for sharing your stories and insights. This project is "our thing" and I hope it lives up to your expectations.

Last but not least, to my new sweetie, Jaime McKenzie. The distractions were worth it because I needed the break. Thank you for showing me that love doesn't have to hurt.

In Jesus' Precious Name,
AMEN

OTHER CONTRIBUTORS

Medical

Barbara Gordon, M.D. Currently a partner in a Brooklyn-based gynecological practice where she services patients in the local community. Attended Brooklyn College for her bachelor's degree and New York Medical College for her medical degree. Her residency in obstetrics and gynecology was completed at the University of New Mexico, Albuquerque, New Mexico, in 1998.

Richard W. Henderson, M.D., F.A.C.O.G. Obstetrician/gynecologist at Saint Francis Hospital based in Wilmington, Delaware.

Henry J. Krebs, III, M.D. Diagnostic and interventional radiologist that specializes in uterine artery embolization for the Radiology Associates of DeKalb, P.C. based in Decatur, GA. E-mail *hkrebs@bell south.net.*

John C. Lipman, M.D. Author of original reports, numerous research papers, and a book. Lectured nationally on uterine fibroid embolization. Also selected to be professional education co-chair by the Society of Cardiovascular and Interventional Radiology for their fibroid embolization task force. Web site *www.micro.yourmd.com*

Dr. Deidre S. Maccannon. Co-director of the National Center of Excellence in Women's Health at the University of Michigan Health

System's Department of Obstetrics and Gynecology. *www.med.umich.edu/obgyn/haltclinic.*

Paula A. McKenzie, M.D. Practices general obstetrics and gynecology at Alexandria WomenCare based in Alexandria, Virginia. She completed medical training at Stanford University and residency at Beth Israel Medical Center.

Debbie Slater. Served as a nurse practitioner for the Ob-Gyn/Women's Health since 1977. Trained by Planned Parenthood of New York City. Currently employed at Woodhull Medical and Mental Health Center and has been working with women with fibroids for twenty-four years.

Cyril Spann, M.D. Associate professor of OB/GYN at Emory University for fifteen years.

Elizabeth Annella Stewart, M.D. Clinical director of the Center for Uterine Fibroids at Brigham and Women's Hospital.

Yvonne S. Thornton, M.D., M.P.H. A perinatal attending physician at St. Luke's Roosevelt Hospital Center in New York. Author of the Pulitzer Prize–nominated book, *The Ditchdigger's Daughters: A Black Family's Astonishing Success Story* (Dafina, $24).

Natural Remedies

Queen Afua. A nationally renowned herbalist, holistic health specialist, and author of *Heal Thyself for Health and Longevity* (A&B, $9.95) and *SACRED WOMAN: A Guide to Healing the Feminine Body, Mind and Spirit* (Ballantine, $28). Runs the Brooklyn-based Heal Thyself health and wellness center.

Sir Abdulla Smithford. Owner of The Perfect Body Health Systems, a Manhattan-based health and wellness center that takes a holistic approach to self-healing.

General Commentary

Empress Zuleika Bes Sekhemet Maat. Dance instructor for Queen Afua's healing center based in Brooklyn, New York. Provided insight on the importance of exercise and dance on healing.

Pastor A. R. Bernard. Spiritual leader for New York Christian Cultural Center based in Brooklyn, New York. The nondenominational church, started more than twenty-two years ago out of a storefront, currently has more than ten thousand members. **(718-272-5150)**

Karima. Brooklyn-based Reiki healer who has been practicing for nearly two years.

Editorial

Leslie E. Royal. A freelance writer and publicist residing in Lithonia, Georgia. Writes for various magazines including *Black Enterprise*, *Upscale,* and *The Atlanta Tribune.* Served as editorial researcher for this book.

Tara Lawrence. Assistant director of training for Woodhull Medical and Mental Health Center. Vice president of Professional Women of Color. Served as editorial researcher for this book.

William Acevedo. Promotions designer for *Black Enterprise* magazine. Developed the illustrations for this book.

Introduction

Great balls of fire! That's the best way I can think of to describe fibroids. Those menacing myomas continued to break down my uterus and burn holes through the depths of my soul.

When I was initially diagnosed with fibroids, Dr. Hobgood (I'll never forget her name) made it seem as if my condition was just a normal part of female development, but that was the furthest thing from the truth. My body was being taken over by some foreign invaders that were on a mission to wreak havoc every step of the way—and they were winning.

At first, my fibroids were nothing more than a menace. I'd be hanging out with my friends and start to experience a leaky-faucet sensation. Upon checking things out, I'd find that I was in the red—literally. And that meant excusing myself so I could get a change of undies and other provisions so I wouldn't end up looking like a bloody mess. It was a big inconvenience, to say the least, but it was also a nuisance that I could manage. At this point, it was only a matter of carrying some "just-in-case" supplies wherever I went. Now, that's not to say that I didn't want a solution. But when I approached my physician about remedying the situation it just didn't appear to be that big of a deal, especially since she'd cancelled my appointments several times to deal with patients that had more important issues—women were giving birth, for God's sake, and all I had were some bothersome fibroids. Maybe I just had to deal with it, I thought.

And I was dealing with it. But the bleeding began to increase on a weekly basis. My menstrual cycle never seemed to end. Sometimes my periods would begin to run into each other and I'd bleed for weeks at a time. I began spending a large portion of my paycheck on what I categorized as "accident wear." These were items that I ended up purchasing at the last minute because of mishaps. I also loaded up on all types of sanitary products, which included any form of "maxi" or "super duper" tampon or napkin that was on the market. The bleeding was affecting me in various ways. I was often dizzy and faint, probably from being so anemic, and I feared that I would pass out in some awkward or dangerous location, so I avoided riding the subway or going out unless it was some work-related activity. I also began to walk funny because the insides of my legs were rubbed raw from the friction that was caused by all of the packing products I had to put on before I got dressed. There was also trouble on the romance front. Since my periods were coming closer together, I blamed PMS for my dwindling libido (sex drive, honey) or claimed it was "that time of the month." He was tired of it and had declared on more than one occasion that he didn't know how much more he could take. I didn't know how much more I could take, either—those fibroids were ruining my life.

Finally some help. My gynecologist prescribed Provera to put the brakes on the bleeding and performed a D&C to try to assess if there were any cancerous cells growing in the lining of my uterus. Now she was talking cancer, even though she initially had said that fibroids were "nothing to worry about." What was going on?

The Provera proved to be a temporary solution for what appeared to be a chronic problem. I decided not to continue as a patient with Dr. Hobgood. Although she was the nicest person you'd ever want to meet, definitely more personable than the other physicians that followed, the cancellations didn't work for me. I needed a physician who was going to make my concerns a priority.

The next few months were followed with a slew of visits to doctors' offices. They all seemed to come up with the same solution: "Try these birth control pills and we'll see what happens." They weren't working.

I finally ended up with a fertility specialist, Dr. F, who reluctantly agreed to surgically remove the fibroids after I wrote him a heart-wrenching letter detailing my experiences. So on August 15, 1997, I had a myolysis, a procedure that shrinks fibroids by blocking their blood supply. My bleeding problems stopped for about two years until the fibroids returned with a vengeance.

Sis, I know it may be hard to believe, but things were actually worse than ever on the second go-around. I was truly living a nightmare. The only time I left the house was to go to work, and that was only when I was wearing three sanitary napkins, one tampon, and a pair of Depends (adult diapers). That packaging secured me for about forty-five minutes. If I didn't make it to my destination in that time period, my clothes were done for the day. A few times I went rushing to the emergency room because I thought I might bleed to death, but I was told that the fibroids were causing the problem and they couldn't do anything to help me. "Come back if you pass out or have some other serious symptom. For now, make an appointment with your gynecologist," they'd say.

By that time, I had seen more than eight gynecologists over a two-year period and there was still no relief in sight—at least without another surgery. My uterus was the size of an eighteen-week pregnancy (that's more than four months). This was critical because a few of the gynecologists that I saw did not want to take the case because of the size of my uterus; their first recommendation would have been a hysterectomy, but that was out of the question for me—I was only twenty-nine years old.

Whether they took my case or not, they all recommended that I have the fibroids removed by myomectomy because my fertility was in jeopardy. But I later found out that my fertility was in jeopardy even if I had the surgery. Women who have a myomectomy run the risk of having an emergency hysterectomy, so doctors insist that patients sign consent forms before going under the knife. "A myomectomy is a very bloody procedure," explains Ifeanyi C. O. Obiakor, M.D., an obstetrician/gynecologist based in Brooklyn, New York. "You may have to perform an emergency hysterectomy to save the patient's life."

Now that was unsettling for me. Not only was I terrified of having another surgery, but the thought of having a hysterectomy (even in an emergency situation) overwhelmed me. So I bowed out of the surgery—twice. I tried to convince myself that things weren't as bad as they seemed. I figured I only had another ten years until menopause so I'd just wait everything out.

In the meanwhile, I stuffed myself into girdles and control-top pantyhose to bind down my growing abdomen. I sat on metal chairs so I wouldn't ruin the few pieces of "untarnished" furniture that I had left. I slept on a bed covered with plastic bags, newspapers, and hospital pads to preserve my mattress and I popped iron pills like candy to keep from passing out from the blood loss. I was handling things—or so I thought.

That was until a friend of mine paid me an extremely rare visit (I never had company at that time) and saw my large belly poking out beneath some of my casual clothes. He didn't know what fibroids were (neither did I until I had to deal with them). But he knew something was terribly wrong, and he helped me summon up the courage to get a solution. On Thursday, August 17, 2000, I finally had a myomectomy.

Although tears streamed down my face all the way to the operating room, I knew there was no other choice for me and I needed a change.

Fortunately, I think my decision was the right one—at least so far. But I think the process that I used to get to my final decision was all wrong. There should have been a better way. Not only for me, but for all women who find themselves in my situation—particularly if they are African American.

Experts say just about every sister you know has fibroids. But you don't have to take their word for it. Just poll the black women in your midst—sister, aunt, coworker, friend, teacher, or confidant—and you'll find that they have fibroids too. Yet the subject gets very little play by health professionals because they feel that fibroids are no big deal. I disagree. I say fibroids are much too costly to ignore. They cost us money in treatments, doctor/emergency room visits, sanitary supplies, and time out of work. According to an article on the Internet (*www.ahrq.gov/clinic/utersumm.htm*), the estimated cost for inpatient fibroid care (primarily surgical) is more than $2 billion in 1997. As Johanna Skilling points out in her book *Fibroids: The Complete Guide to Taking Charge of Your Physical, Emotional, and Sexual Well-Being* (Marlowe & Company, $15.95), fibroids also have a host of costs that don't involve money. When fibroids start causing a ruckus in your body, your relationships, sexual pleasure, physical well-being, and emotional health suffer. And if you're an African American woman, the price that you're forced to pay is much higher than for your white counterparts.

Will reading this book help you eliminate all of the consequences that lie ahead of you as a fibroid sufferer? Absolutely not. Much of what we know about what causes fibroids as well as how to treat them is based on theory. These ideas aren't necessarily facts. At the same time, the theories highlighted here may help you develop a treatment plan that proves true for you, and that's all that matters. Use the exercises at the end of each chapter to help you evaluate your options, gather your medical history, select a medical practitioner, track your progress, and better prepare you for your next doctor's visit. Complete each of them and put them in a safe place so that you can dig them up when it's time for your next doctor's appointment. Also, don't overlook the stories of the numerous women who know exactly what you're going through. These "sistahs" not only have tales to tell but can also offer insight on the resources that are available to you and how you can best use them. Finally, I hope you'll use the dialogue in this book as a platform for you to share your own story with others. If you really want to inspire doctors and the rest of the medical community to find better ways to treat fibroid sufferers, then you must sound the alarm about your dissatisfaction with the current system and support other sisterfriends who are meeting similar challenges. Fibroids, whether we like it or not, have come to be "a sistah thing," so it's up to each of us to do something about it.

1

Why Me?

Understanding Fibroids in Black Women

This wasn't an ordinary Saturday. You see, my weekly library visit was cut short due to an unexpected guest. Well, it wasn't actually a guest; to call it that makes it sound like the visitor was welcomed—and there was nothing further from the truth. It was old Aunt Flo. She dropped by right when I was thumbing through the 600s for a book on money management. I was trying to get my financial house in order and Auntie dropped in to shake things up.

Prior to that, her visits were like clockwork, so the surprise caught me without my usual welcoming supplies. Of course, Grand Army Plaza wasn't at all accommodating. So I made a mad dash for the nearest grocery store and concluded that the incident must have been some kind of a fluke. Boy was I wrong, that was just her premiere. Miss Thang popped in while I was at work, riding home on the train, kicking it on a date, and any other inappropriate times she could find. Aunt Flo was on point. Every time she made an appearance it was much more memorable than the last. And she was always the center of attention since she muscled her way into situations that were sure to result in pure humiliation and embarrassment.

—Monique Brown, Age 32, Magazine Editor

Girlfriend, if you're anywhere near your late twenties or early thirties, you've probably had some encounter with uterine fibroids. Either you've been bothered by them or someone you know has—maybe both.

First off, let's examine the word *fibroid.* Despite the fact that it has crept into everyday use, the term is a misnomer. Fibroids are not derived from fibrous tissue, as the word implies, but are developed from muscle cells. So the more accurate yet less commonly used medical term *leiomyoma (leio* means smooth, *my* means muscle, and *oma* means growth or tumor) is more appropriate.[1] Other medical terms include *fibromyoma, leiomyofibroma,* and *myoma.* But the simple term, and the one we'll be using for the most part, is *fibroid.* I just thought it was important that you be familiar with other terms should you encounter them.

So you know what to call them, but the real question is "What are fibroids?" By definition fibroids are "benign tumors of muscle cell origin found in any tissue that contains smooth muscle."[2] That's right, fibroids can develop in muscle tissue throughout the body, but they are most commonly found in the uterus. In fact, fibroids are the most common growth in the uterus or pelvic region. They vary widely by location and size. For example, they can develop on the surface of the uterus, within the walls, in the uterine cavity, or in two or all three locations. They also vary widely by size and number. They can remain as small as a pea or grow as large as a full-term pregnancy. Some women have a single fibroid, while others have numerous ones. In short, fibroid tumors are about as varied as the women who have them.

Now, if you're like most people, the word *tumor* may cause some alarm because you associate it with cancer. But relax, fibroids are always benign, or noncancerous. Experts report that the incidence of leiomyosarcoma, an extremely rare form of malignant tumor of the uterine muscle, occurs in only 0.1 percent to 0.7 percent of women diagnosed with fibroid tumors. Women over sixty years of age who are admitted to a hospital with the diagnosis of fibroids are ten times more likely to be found to have leiomyosarcoma than a woman who is forty or younger. But even that's an overstatement, because many women don't even know they have fibroids so they are never diagnosed. In fact, most gynecologists never see leiomyosarcoma during the life of their practice.[3]

Still, the presence of fibroids does indicate an abnormal growth of tissue in the uterus. The strange thing is that this abnormality is so common that almost every woman you know probably has them, whether they know it or not. According to the Center for Uterine Fibroids at Boston's Brigham and Women's Hospital, 80 percent of all women have fibroids.[4] Traditionally, fibroids were estimated to be present in 25 to 50 percent of women of childbearing age, with the greatest prevalence among women in their thirties and forties.[5] However, recent research suggests that fibroids may exist in as many as three out of four females, indicating that 25 to 80 million American women have fibroids.[6]

Sisters are fibroids' biggest victims. They are three to nine times more common in African American women than in the general population.[7] Fibroids in black women also tend to be larger, grow more quickly, and be more numerous than in other groups, according to a study supported in part by the Agency for Health Care Policy and Research.[8] So they're more likely to experience severe symptoms from them. In addition, black women tend to develop problems from fibroids at an earlier age than other groups. In a study conducted by the University of Maryland School of Medicine,[9] researchers found that of the 409 black women who had a hysterectomy at twenty-eight Maryland hospitals, 89 percent had fibroids compared to 59 percent of the 836 white female patients. In addition, the black women with fibroids averaged thirty-eight years old, while their white counterparts averaged forty-two years old. The sisters were also younger when they underwent their hysterectomy, averaging forty-two years old while white women averaged forty-five years old. These results seem pretty consistent with other findings. According to Francis L. Hutchins, M.D., on Fibroidzone.com, it's not unusual for a black woman in her mid- to late twenties to be diagnosed with these tumors. "Some African-American women have had *myomectomies* (surgical removal of fibroids from the uterus) as young as 17 years of age!"[10]

But as with everything else, knowledge is the key to unlocking a world of possible solutions. The more you know, the better you'll be able to manage your situation and choose a strategy that's right for you. This chapter offers theories explaining why fibroids occur more frequently in African American women than in other groups, takes a close look at where fibroids occur in the uterus, answers questions relating to our own physical health, and highlights a physician's checklist so you can gain a clearer understanding of your fibroid condition.

HERE'S THE UNDENIABLE TRUTH

Since much of the information surrounding fibroids remains a mystery, it's important that you familiarize yourself with the available facts. Here's the 4-1-1 on fibroids:

- Fibroids typically grow in multiples of about five to seven.
- Fibroids by definition are not cancerous.
- Females do not develop fibroids prior to the onset of menstruation.

- Fibroids do not have to be treated by hysterectomy.
- Fibroids do not always cause symptoms.
- A large proportion of women don't even know they have fibroids.
- Fibroids are more common in black women than in women in other racial groups.
- Fibroids reduce in size at the onset of menopause.
- Having uterine fibroids does not mean you have a tendency for increased "fibrocystic" changes in other areas such as the breast.

That's the long and short of what we already know about fibroids, everything else is all theory. That's not to say that the theories are false; it just means that there isn't enough scientific information available to convert those theories to facts. So you have to decide what information makes sense to you and use it to remedy your condition. But we've got a little ways to go before you start pinpointing a plan of action; first I'm going to attempt to answer the question that has been on your mind ever since you've been diagnosed with fibroids: "Why me?"

FIBROIDS AND AFRICAN AMERICAN WOMEN

The word fibroids entered my vocabulary as subtly as the mass grew in my body. More and more I found myself talking about it, thinking about it, fearing it. In my body now grew "something." Some matter that fed on my blood, reacted to my increasing stress level, and even supposedly responded to my diet. When I asked my doctor why this was happening or what I could do to get rid of them, she gave a short, noncommittal response. "No one knows why most black women have them," she said flatly. "We'll just have to wait and see."

Her answer did nothing to alleviate my concerns.

—Danette Jordan, Age 36

Even though fibroids are a common occurrence among women, particularly in women of African descent, very little is known about why they develop and why some women never seem to get them. As you might imagine, there is even less information available about why black women are more susceptible than other groups. Still, there are some theories as to why black women are the leading candidates for uterine fibroids. Here's what might be causing your fibroids:

TOO MANY POUNDS TIPPING THE SCALE[11]

According to Ziba Kashef, "excess weight may contribute to fibroids because body fat, particularly fat around the abdomen, produces estrogen." Estrogen is a leading agent in the development of fibroids.

"The majority of black women are overweight to some degree, which may in part explain the high prevalence of fibroids, and severity of related symptoms, in our community," Kashef writes in her book

USDA Suggested Weights for Adults

Height*	Weight**	
	Age 19–34 years	Age >35 years old
5'0"	97–128	108–138
5'1"	101–132	111–143
5'2"	104–137	115–148
5'3"	107–141	119–152
5'4"	111–146	122–157
5'5"	114–150	126–162
5'6"	118–155	130–167
5'7"	121–160	134–172
5'8"	125–164	138–178
5'9"	129–169	142–183
5'10"	132–174	146–188
5'11"	136–179	151–194
6'0"	140–184	155–199

*Height is without shoes.
**Weight is without clothes. The heavier weights generally apply to men, who typically have greater bone mass and muscle than women.
Source: U.S. Dept. of Agriculture and U.S. Dept. of Health and Human Services, *Nutrition and Your Health: Dietary Guidelines for Americans*, 3d ed. (Washington, D.C.: U.S. Government Printing Office, 1990) as printed in *Women's Bodies, Women's Wisdom* (Bantam, 1998).

Like a Natural Woman: The Black Woman's Guide to Alternative Healing (Kensington, $15). According to the Third National Health and Nutrition Examination Survey, half of all African American women are obese, exceeding their ideal weight by 10 to 20 percent. This suggests that black women need to rethink their eating habits because fat gets converted to estrogen, the main contributor to fibroid development.

WHAT YOU EAT

According to Kashef, "a diet high in fat and processed foods may be a major factor in the creation of fibroids." In Kashef's book, Dr. Jewel Pookrum, an Atlanta-based holistic gynecologist, points out that the African American woman's high-meat diet puts undue stress on the liver, preventing it from properly breaking down fat and protein and from removing excess estrogen from the blood.

Bridgette York of *Fibroid News* also suggests that the type of food African American women eat largely influences the development of fibroids. She says black women's bodies don't react well to Western diets, which largely consist of substances that are high in saturated fats, meats, and dairy products. York says these ingredients, which can mimic the increased estrogen that occurs during pregnancy or menstruation, stimulate cells in the uterus and breast to reproduce. She adds, "The excess estrogen caused by diets makes your body think it's preparing to implant an egg 28 days a month."

THOSE CRAZY HORMONES

"No one knows exactly what causes [fibroids]. It's clear, though, that excessive estrogen levels makes fibroids worse."[12] Excessive estrogen causes uterine cells to be overstimulated, and that's not good. Fibroids begin with a single cell that somehow goes haywire; they are given the wrong signals about how they are supposed to grow.

When estrogen behaves properly, it shoots a message over to the ovaries when it's time to release an egg and causes the lining of the uterus to thicken during ovulation. This environment makes it easier for a fertilized egg to attach itself to the womb. If you become pregnant, the production of estrogen decreases and progesterone kicks in to help the fertilized egg absorb nutrients. But if the egg doesn't become fertilized, the estrogen and progesterone levels drop, the lining breaks down, and you have your period. However, some women maintain high levels of estrogen throughout the menstrual cycle, and the cells in the uterus become overstimulated and may eventually develop into fibroids.

Excess estrogen can also be caused by long periods of exposure to it. Since black women typically start menstruating a year earlier than their white counterparts, they are exposed to estrogen over longer periods in their lifetime and have a greater tendency to live in polluted areas where they're in contact with environmental chemicals that may mimic hormones. The *Alternative Medicine Guide to Women's Health Series* points out ten other factors that could contribute to a hormonal imbalance:

- eating too many foods that have synthetic hormones added to them such as eggs, meat, and dairy products;
- ingesting herbs that behave like estrogen such as black cohosh, damiana, and licorice;
- using high-estrogen birth control pills;
- chronic constipation, which prevents the proper elimination of estrogen;
- being exposed to environmental toxins that mimic estrogen such as pesticides;
- exposure to radiation;
- use of menopausal hormonal supplements;
- poorly functioning thyroid gland;
- an excessive occurrence of menstruation without ovulation;
- recurring stress.

For the most part, it's been found that women with fibroids have normal estrogen levels. What occurs is that their uterine cells go through a change that causes them to use up (or metabolize) excessive amounts of estrogen. The relationship between fibroid growth and estrogen is further supported when we look at girls prior to menstruation and postmenopausal women. Neither of these groups produce fibroids because they do not produce estrogen.

Some experts say that progesterone[13] also contributes to fibroid growth, and there are clinical studies to support this theory. For example, it was found that fibroids increase in size in response to synthetic progesterones. In addition, fibroids treated with progesterone show more growth than those without this type of therapy. Further, fibroids tend to shrink in response to the antiprogesterone agent RU-486.

Other hormones such as prolactin (PRL) and growth hormone (GH) have also been fingered for promoting fibroid growth, but those theories are inconclusive.

BEING STRESSED OUT

Some experts associate fibroids with a psychosocial disorder. According to Dr. Pookrum, fibroid sufferers share certain characteristics which she profiles as the "F personality." She says they have ambivalence regarding motherhood, have concerns about their romantic relationships, are dissatisfied with their work, and lack self-nurturing. Their frustrations manifest themselves in the form of uterine fibroids. Dr. Grace Cornish, author of 10 Good Choices That Empower Black Women's Lives, agrees that the stress level among African American women has caused physical dysfunctions. She points out that the American Heart Association reported that black women are three to five times more likely to suffer or die from cardiovascular problems than their white counterparts. She writes, "Black women are especially stressed out because they are burdened with negative images and false standards, and they have had to keep their mouths shut about their pain for far too long."

Another theory linking stress and fibroids suggests that a high stress level causes us to tense parts of our body, including the pelvic muscles.[14] This prohibits proper blood flow to and from the uterus, which also prevents toxins from being sufficiently expelled. Uterine fibroids are the result.

BAD RELATIONSHIPS

Having toxic people in your life can manifest itself in various ways, and some experts feel fibroids are by-products of this emotional trauma. According to an article on Voice of Women (*www.voiceof women.com/articles/fibroids.html*), women develop fibroids when they have problems with their relationship to sex, work, physical desire, and people. Observes the author of this article, "In reviewing my history and struggle with fibroids, I discovered that when I was experiencing relationship issues the fibroids grew." I noticed that as well.

Queen Afua, a holistic practitioner, herbalist, and author, has observed this in her patients. "We go from one relationship to the next but we haven't resolved the previous relationship," she notes. "So we keep building up all of these womb hurts and womb traumas. . . . We are our relationships and that's what grows disease and tumors."

TAKING AFTER MOM

Did you ask anybody else in your family if they had fibroids? Fibroids are considered familial. I bet if you chatted with your mother, aunts, cousins, and other relatives, you'd probably find that they also suffer from these menacing myomas. That's because there appears to be a close relationship between fibroids and heredity,[15] according to Ziba Kashef. Henry J. Krebs, III, M.D., an interventional radiologist specializing in artery embolization, agrees. He's found that "seven out of 10 patients have family members such as a mother, daughter or sister with fibroids." But the fact that you and other family members have fibroids in common may have more to do with the habits you inherited—such as food consumption, lack of exercise, and techniques for handling stress—than the genes you got.

Although there still hasn't been any concrete evidence to prove that fibroids are indeed hereditary, many experts say their hunch is based on years of observation. "Chromosome 12" seems to be the gene that contains the misinformation that triggers fibroids, states Dr. Deidre S. Maccannon, co-director of the National Center of Excellence in Women's Health at the University of Michigan. "We've known for quite some time that there is a genetic predisposition [in fibroid development]," adds Maccannon.

Dr. Elizabeth Annella Stewart agrees. The clinical director of the Center for Uterine Fibroids at Brigham and Women's Hospital says there is an indication that fibroids seem to move throughout generations. "Lab evidence suggests that the disruption of a certain gene called Hmgic appears to be associated with fibroids," Stewart explains. "We are also researching some genes due to hereditary and some environmental exposure."

Talk to Mom and Other Female Relatives

You've heard the saying "Momma knows best." Well, her insight may be particularly relevant where fibroids are concerned. There is some indication that fibroids have a similar pattern among family members. So if your mother, grandmothers, aunts, and other female relatives have fibroids, you should gather information about their experiences. But you've got to talk to them first. Here's how you can start:

Have a one-to-one chat over tea, brunch, or whatever. Maybe you've heard that Grandma, Aunt Sue, or Cousin Jane was treated for "female problems" and you've got a sneaky suspicion that fibroids may have been the culprit. Find out for yourself. If you think they won't feel comfortable dishing out the details in a group setting, see if they'll give you the skinny in private. First, let them know that you're trying to gather some family health information. Openly express your concerns about fibroids and share your experiences. Tell them that you want to know if they've ever had problems with fibroids because research indicates that fibroids may run in families. Then promise to keep whatever they tell you under wraps and stick to your word.

Some questions to ask:

- Do you have fibroids?

- When were you diagnosed?

- How old were you when you were diagnosed?

- How large are they currently?

- Do you suffer symptoms from them?

- What methods did they use to diagnose them (ultrasound, MRI, etc.)?

- What options did your doctor offer?

- How did you choose to treat them?

- Why did you make that decision?

- Did you suffer side effects from the treatment?

- Did you get a second opinion?

- How are your fibroids doing today?

- What advice would you offer other women with fibroids?

Once you've gotten the information, organize it in a journal or file. Then compare their answers to these questions with your own responses. Do you see any similarities? Share your findings with your gynecologist.

ENTERING MOTHERHOOD

So you're having a baby? That means your body is producing higher levels of estrogen. And as we learned earlier, estrogen can stimulate fibroid growth. As a result, you may find that your fibroids are getting larger and growing a lot faster since you've gotten pregnant; other fibroid sufferers report that as well. In fact, most women indicated a tendency for their fibroids to increase during pregnancy and shrink after delivery. But as to whether their findings were accurate, that's still up for discussion. A 1988 study that closely monitored pregnant women with fibroids reported that 80 percent remained the same size during the course of gestation with only a small portion actually growing (20 percent).[16] But even if you're one of the women that experience accelerated fibroid growth during pregnancy, your myomas will return to their prepregnancy size after you deliver your bundle of joy.

DELAYING MOTHERHOOD

You probably think this is crazy. Does this mean that your choice to delay having children until you're emotionally and financially ready could be responsible for your fibroid condition? Not exactly. Researchers can't tell whether being childless causes fibroids or if having fibroids results in fertility problems that hinder pregnancy. It's one of those "which came first, the chicken or the egg" scenarios. In any case, experts find that women who have never had a baby tend to be more fibroid-prone than women who do have children.

GETTING OLDER

Among the risk factors is being between the ages of forty and forty-five. Overall, fibroids are estimated in up to 25 percent of women over the age of thirty and in nearly 40 percent of women after the age of forty.[17] At one time this wasn't necessarily seen as a bad thing, because this was at the end of a woman's reproductive years. The majority of women at this age were finished having children, so they could choose to have a hysterectomy or deal with the symptoms until they reached menopause, a time when fibroids shrink on their own.

However, as a larger proportion of today's women delay having children, fibroids have become a more serious issue for women in this age group. In addition, it has been found that removing the uterus (known as a hysterectomy) can cause serious complications. Twenty-five to 50

Fast Fibroid Facts for Sistahs

- Black women are from three to nine times more likely than white women to have fibroids.

- Black women are typically diagnosed with more myomas than their white counterparts.

- Black women are commonly diagnosed with fibroids at a younger age than women in other groups.

- Black women fibroid sufferers tend to have more symptoms than women in other groups.

- Black women are overrepresented among patients that have hysterectomies for fibroids.

Source: Women's Health
http://www.ahcpr.gov/research/nov96/ra1.htm

percent of women who have had a hysterectomy experience one or more complications such as pelvic pain, weight gain, ovarian failure, depression, or other difficulties.[18] As with any operation, there's also the small, but real, risk of death. Women who have had a hysterectomy with the removal of the ovaries also experience the discomforts associated with menopause such as hot flashes and vaginal dryness.

WHAT'S UP WITH THE GRIEF?

It's bad enough when you find out you have these invaders, but when they start to cause you grief that's when your concerns mount. Sis, you're not alone. Once I realized that fibroids were behind my discomfort I wondered why I had to deal with this type of drama, especially when I found out that a large proportion of women never even know they have fibroids. Then I discovered that there are two main reasons that a fibroid can wreak havoc: size and location. According to an article in *Ebony* magazine, "The size of a fibroid has everything to do with the symptoms a woman experiences and the treatment options available to her. The general rule of thumb is that the smaller the fibroid, the easier it is to treat." So if your doctor tells you that your fibroid is the size of an orange, you're in a much better position than I was because mine could be compared to a large melon or a five-month pregnancy. That was the size of it.

Another reason your fibroids may be causing you discomfort may have to do with their location, location, location. Fibroids get their names and are identified according to where they are located in the uterus. There are three primary types:

Type: Intramural
Other Names: Interstitial
Description: Located within the uterus walls, intramural fibroids are the most common types of myomas. The ball-shaped masses can alter the cavity of the uterus and as they grow larger may cause heavy bleeding and cramping during your period. On the other hand, if you have small intramural fibroids you may be symptom-free.

Type: Subserosal
Other Names: serosal, subserous, extramural, or subperitoneal

Sizing up your fibroids

Your doctor may describe your fibroid as related to the size of a pregnant uterus, a technique that probably came about because a layman (or woman) might mistakenly confuse large fibroids with an actual pregnancy. Or maybe your fibroid was compared to the size of a piece of fruit or other objects such as a tennis ball. Regardless of the term used, find out how your fibroids measure up by getting your physician to discuss them in terms that you can understand.

Size of Uterus	Fruit	Pregnancy Talk
Normal	Small pear	N/A
8–10 weeks or 2 months	Orange	You may not even know you have fibroids.
12 weeks or 5 months	Grapefruit	Your uterus has grown to the level of the pubic bone.
16 weeks	Melon	Your fibroid uterus has grown to the midpoint between your pubic bone and your belly button. Feeling a little bloated, your enlarged uterus may cause your clothes to fit a little snug.
20–22 weeks	Pineapple	At this point, you don't need your doctor to tell you that your fibroids are large, because your fibroid uterus has grown up to the level of your belly button. This is the size of a uterus of someone who is approximately five months pregnant.
28 weeks or 7 months	Pumpkin	Your abdomen is substantially enlarged and you look pregnant.
40 weeks	Watermelon	If you were expecting, you'd be ready to deliver. But hopefully you've taken action before now. This is the size of a full-term pregnancy.

Source: Nelson H. Stringer, M.D., *Uterine Fibroids: What Every Woman Needs to Know.*

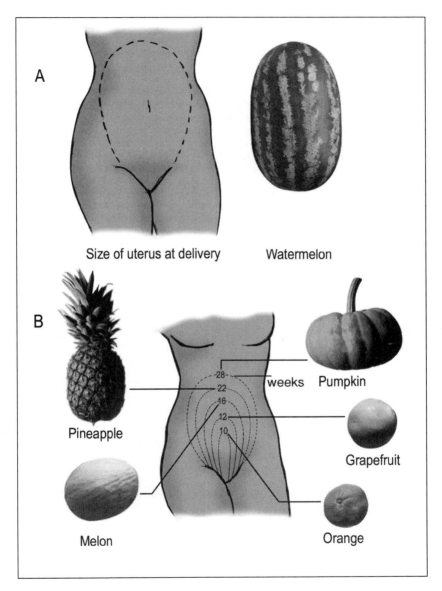

How Large is Your Fibroid?

Description: Located or attached to the outside body of the uterus. The subserosal fibroid grows from the outer walls of the uterus and may apply pressure to the other organs such as the bladder and ureter. When they enlarge, they can cause a swelling of your abdomen that could cause you to look and feel pregnant.

Forms: Pedunculated fibroids are attached to a stalk. They hang outside of the uterus much like a piece of fruit on a branch. These forms of subserosal fibroids can protrude from the uterus, causing the abdomen to appear swollen, or they may attach themselves to other organs or pelvic muscles. If they outgrow their blood supply, they usurp blood from other organs in close proximity, this is why they are also referred to as parasitic leiomyomas.

Sessile fibroids are embedded in the wall of the womb and can also cause bloating or swelling.

Type: Submucous

Other Names: N/A

Description: Located under the uterus' lining, submucous fibroids are rare. They occur in approximately 5 percent of women.[19] However, when they are present they can wreak havoc as they interfere with the development of the lining in the uterus. Women with these types of fibroids may experience heavy bleeding, longer periods, and pain. Submucous fibroids are the most common culprits when it's determined that a fibroid is interfering with a pregnancy because they can take up space in the endometrium and prevent the fertilized egg from attaching to the uterus.

Forms: Like serosal fibroids, submucous fibroids come in two forms: sessile or pendunculated, which are both intracavity fibroids. Sessile fibroids are attached. While pendunculated fibroids "hang into the cavity like a light fixture dangling from the ceiling"[20] and can protrude right through the cervical canal. A specific condition related to the pendunculated fibroid is called torsion. That's when the dangling fibroid twists, causing excruciating pain.

The rarest types of myomas, cervical fibroids, are located at the opening of the cervix. Although they occur in less than 1 percent of women,[21] when they exist they can cause interference when a woman is trying to conceive or cause problems during delivery. The most common type of fibroids, intramural or subserosal, are actually hybrids and may not be classified as one pure type of fibroid, according to Carla Dionne in her book, *Sex, Lies & the Truth About Uterine Fibroids*

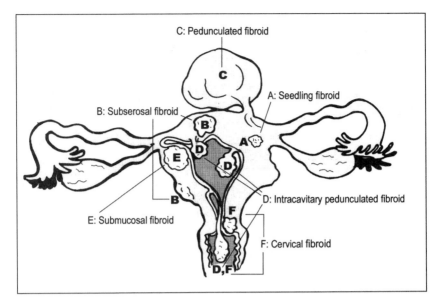

Types of Fibroids

(Avery, $14.95). Still, finding out where your fibroids are located may give you some insight on how your physician plans to treat them, so ask about the location, location, location.

So now you know more about the critters behind your discomfort. Even if your doctor hasn't told you which type of fibroids you have, you may be able to guess based on the symptoms you experience. Still, it's best to gather as much information as you can so you can get the facts on your own fibroids.

MY MYOMAS AND ME

Girlfriend, I can tell you all the facts in the world about how fibroids generally affect us sisters, but everybody's experience is different. Only you know how your fibroids are affecting your body. Below make a list of all of the troubles you think your fibroids are causing such as pelvic

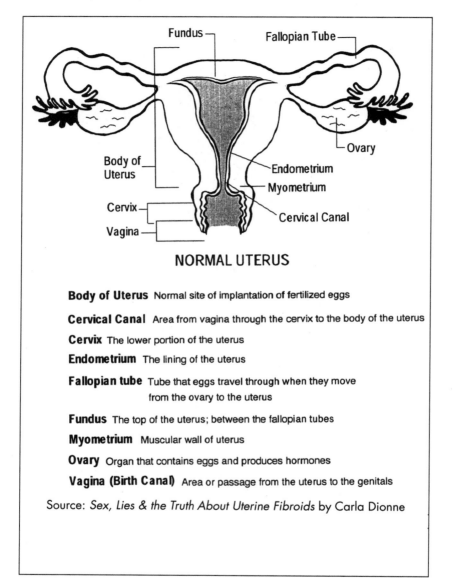

NORMAL UTERUS

Body of Uterus Normal site of implantation of fertilized eggs

Cervical Canal Area from vagina through the cervix to the body of the uterus

Cervix The lower portion of the uterus

Endometrium The lining of the uterus

Fallopian tube Tube that eggs travel through when they move
                   from the ovary to the uterus

Fundus The top of the uterus; between the fallopian tubes

Myometrium Muscular wall of uterus

Ovary Organ that contains eggs and produces hormones

Vagina (Birth Canal) Area or passage from the uterus to the genitals

Source: *Sex, Lies & the Truth About Uterine Fibroids* by Carla Dionne

pain, abnormal bleeding, cramps, fatigue, anemia, urinary and bowel problems, infertility, and any other annoyances that come to mind. Then take this list to your gynecologist and discuss your concerns. The next chapter will tell you just how much of a menace fibroids can be if you're one of the unlucky ones that suffer symptoms from them.

The trouble with my fibroids is:

_____

_____

_____

_____

2 Sizing Up Your Symptoms

Looking at How Fibroids Affect Your Body

Girl, you're talking about DRAMA! I experienced it monthly for about three years of my life. My fibroid started out the size of a green olive in the front wall of my uterus. At first it caused me to have VERY, VERY, VERY heavy bleeding and my periods lasted from seven to ten days every twenty-eight days like clockwork. It was accompanied by excruciating pain on the first and second days of my period. In fact, I was in so much pain that my legs would go numb. I was forced to wear black pants or skirts when I had my period—even in the summertime—because I would bleed through anything I had on. At this point in time I was prescribed Tylenol 3 with codeine to deal with my horrible pain! But it didn't work. When I woke up the next day, I went straight to my doctor's office doubled over in pain.

—Faatimah Kim Monique Smith-Murray, Age 31
Founder of "The Children's Garden, Their Place to Blossom and Grow"
Child Day Care Provider in Harlem

If you're one of the unlucky sistahs that's going through some fibroid drama, it may be hard to believe that "most fibroids do not cause any symptoms and do not require treatment."[1] Research has found that only 20 to 50 percent of the women that have fibroids actually suffer symptoms from them.[2] These estimates are probably exaggerated because the majority of women, sisters included, never even know that they have fibroids and won't want to do a thing about them when they find out. In most cases, fibroids are discovered during a woman's routine GYN exam. In fact, existing myomas may even grow to a startling size before a physician detects them. If that happened to you, your doctors may have suggested that the two of you just observe the growth of your fibroid over the next six months to a year. That's pretty sound advice since there's nothing dangerous about fibroids just hanging around as long as they're not causing trouble. The problem is, the bigger they get, the more likely they are to cause you grief.

Just what kind of havoc can a troubling fibroid wreak? Almost anything you can imagine. Believe me, I know. I was one of the unlucky ladies that experienced the majority of the symptoms that plague fibroid sufferers. Although fibroids are most commonly known for causing bleeding and pelvic pressure,[3] there are a wealth of other symptoms fibroid sufferers may experience. Other complaints include heavy periods, bleeding in between periods, anemia, fatigue, distortion of the abdomen, frequent urination, constipation, painful intercourse, cramping, varicose veins, premature labor, infertility, miscarriage, and depression.

For us, fibroids can be particularly troublesome. "Estimates show that fibroids will cause symptoms in half of all Black women by age 50, compared to 30 percent of White women."[4] Take the study conducted by the University of Maryland School of Medicine; its researchers found that black women were more likely than white women to suffer symptoms from fibroids and experience more severe reactions. For example, black women in the study were more likely than their white counterparts to have seven or more fibroids (57 percent vs. 36 percent), to have severe pelvic pain (59 percent vs. 41 percent), and to be anemic (56 percent vs. 38 percent).[5]

So, girl, if you thought your mind was playing tricks on you and your uterus, that may be the furthest thing from the truth. As your fibroids start to elbow their way around in the struggle for more space, they may be raising quite a ruckus and this disturbance could be causing you discomfort. In this chapter, we take a close look at how fibroids may make you feel and how you can handle the nuisance in the short term. If you're ready to size up your symptoms, check out these complaints:

BLEEDING

I had never even heard of fibroid tumors until I started bleeding heavily. My periods were usually three days, but when I developed the fibroids, they went up to ten days. I started feeling uncomfortable going to meetings at work and I started looking behind me to make sure no spots were left on the chairs. I also had to put plastic on my car seats and always checked out my clothes to make sure they weren't stained.

— Norma Chappell, Freelance Writer and Publicist

Excessive bleeding, experienced by 30 percent of women with fibroids, is the most common complaint. It's also "the most immediate, the most visible, and the most physical symptom women with fibroids can have," according to Johanna Skilling, author of *Fibroids: The Complete Guide to Taking Charge of Your Physical, Emotional, and Sexual Well-Being* (Marlowe $24.95). Abnormal bleeding may start during your periods; you may have noticed that they are heavier than usual (menorrhagia) and are lasting for more days (metrorrhagia) than usual. Some women, in fact, bleed almost constantly (menometrorrhagia).[6]

Bleeding Terms to Remember

- Amenorrhea: No period at all for more than six months.

- Ovulatory bleeding: A normal period that comes every twenty-one to thirty-five days without passage of large chunks of clots, lasting no more than eight days.

- Hypomenorrhea: Light or scanty periods that last the normal number of days.

- Intermenstrual bleeding: Also referred to as breakthrough bleeding. Occurs between periods. You may have experienced this type of bleeding if you missed a birth control pill. Bleeding of variable amounts that occur between regular periods.

- Metrorrhagia: Bleeding irregularly at frequent intervals. The quantity of bleeding may vary (from heavy to spotting). It may be bleeding in between periods or periods lasting more than seven days.

- Menorrhagia: Excessive bleeding that is heavier, that may be associated with the passage of large chunks of clots, and may last longer than your normal period.

- Oligomenorrhea: Long gaps between periods that are greater than thirty-five days.

- Polymenorrhea: Bleeding occurring at regular intervals but less than twenty-one days. For example, you'd have this condition if your period came every two weeks.

There are several reasons that fibroids cause heavy bleeding. A major cause is related to the type of fibroids that you have in your uterus. Fibroids housed in the walls of your uterus prevent it from contracting properly. Your uterus is a muscle that has the unique ability to squeeze the blood vessels shut during your period; these contractions may cause you to feel cramps during that time of the month. When a fibroid is present, however, it may keep the blood vessels from closing completely, and this allows you to lose more blood. Another theory proposes that when the blood vessels that feed into a fibroid become excessively enlarged, the body's normal blood clotting function becomes ineffective. Lastly, a protein that reduces muscle tone in smooth-muscle cells[7] can cause the uterus to relax and allow blood vessels to bleed more freely than normal.

Submucous fibroids, for example, are a type of myoma that grows underneath the lining of the uterus (endometrium) and are almost always identified as the prime suspect when excessive bleeding is present. It makes sense that submucous fibroids would be blamed for this symptom because as these tumors grow, they cause the lining of the uterus to stretch, thin out, and disfigure—all of these conditions cause bleeding. However, only 5 percent of fibroids are believed to be submucous, and excessive bleeding is present in 30 percent of fibroid sufferers. The numbers don't add up.[8]

So how do you know when your bleeding is cause for alarm? Experts say you shouldn't lose more than 80 milliliters (two to three ounces or a quarter of a cup) during your period. In simpler terms, if you find yourself having to change your pad at least once an hour or passing large chunks of clots, that's not a good sign.[9] Excessive blood loss could indicate medical conditions other than fibroids such as polyps, hormonal changes, an overgrowth of the lining of the uterus, and on rare occasions precancer or cancer of the uterus.[10] In addition, your body may be unable to replace the blood cells that you've lost fast enough and that could result in anemia, indicating an iron deficiency which could result in shortness of breath, fatigue, and dizziness as well as other symptoms.

Check the Signs

Could you be anemic? Blood level can be monitored in two ways, either by the amount of hemoglobin present, which is measured in grams, or by hematocrit, which is measured in percentages. According to Dr. Elizabeth Annella Stewart of Boston, anemia is indicated when your level of hemoglobin (the protein that carries oxygen to the blood) is low and your level of hematocrit, the percentage of red blood cells in whole blood, is low. You're considered anemic if your hemoglobin is less than 12 or if your hematocrit is less than 35 percent.

How often do you change your fully soaked pad or tampon? If you're soaking through a pad every hour, then that should be a cause for concern. In a period of five days, you should use about a box of pads.

What was your last hemoglobin reading? A normal level is 12 to 15 grams.

Do you have the signs of anemia? Some signs are that you often feel tired, feel drained, crave ice, or have difficulty climbing stairs. Symptoms are generally worse after your period, before your body has a chance to rebuild your blood count.

ANEMIA

Anemia occurs when your body doesn't have enough iron in your blood. When your body lacks iron, it isn't able to efficiently process oxygen. As a result, you may begin to feel weak, tired, and lightheaded. In addition, anemia also causes heart palpitations because the lack of oxygen causes the heart to beat faster and can lower your body's resistance to disease.

Physicians can tell you whether or not you have anemia from the results of two tests—hemoglobin and hematocrit. The hemoglobin test measures the weight of the number of molecules in the blood that carry oxygen.[11] A normal level is 12 to 15 grams per liter or a quart of blood. The hematocrit measures the ratio of red blood cells to plasma which should be about 35 percent to 50 percent. Red blood cells carry oxygen. Within the normal range, the higher the proportion of red blood cells, the better the reading.

Girlfriend, if you're experiencing heavy bleeding from your fibroids, start keeping a record of your hemoglobin and hematocrit levels after each testing. A hemoglobin of less than 10 grams or a hematocrit of less than 30 percent indicates that your anemia requires treatment. As a first step, your doctor will probably prescribe iron pills to help build up your blood count. In addition, birth control pills may be suggested as a means to regulate your bleeding and improve anemia. However, if your condition does worsen, you can expect your physician to offer the surgical removal of your fibroids as the next alternative.

FATIGUE

Your fibroids may be sucking the energy right out of your system causing you to feel downright pooped. I've felt the same way too, and experts offer several explanations:

A fibroid's survival depends on a large blood supply. They're using up blood that your body may need for other functions to work properly. Also, if you're losing an excessive amount of blood and suffering from anemia, that could be contributing to your fatigue. And if you've been worrying about how you're going to tackle those menacing myomas, this distress could also be wearing you out. Lastly, large fibroids may also add a few pounds, so carrying the extra weight could produce a tired feeling. My fibroids caused my uterus to be the size of a five-month pregnancy. Once I shed those four large fibroids, my dress size went from a size seven to a size four and I came out of surgery about eight pounds lighter. What a relief!

PELVIC PRESSURE

What symptoms do most fibroid sufferers complain about? You probably know firsthand that irregular bleeding and pelvic pressure are the most common complaints heard from women with fibroids. We've already talked about why fibroids cause bleeding, but the pressure you may be feeling is caused by the mere size of them. As your womb enlarges, it can press on other organs such as the intestines and the bladder. As your uterus grows, your bladder becomes smaller, and that may cause you to make more trips to the ladies' room even though you'll find you only have to release a small amount of urine once you get there. You may also experience urinary incontinence, a condition that causes you to leak urine when you laugh, sneeze, or exert yourself. Your enlarged uterus could also press against the ureters, the passageways that transport urine from your kidneys, but this is uncommon. In extreme cases, however, a backup of urine could cause kidney infection or damage. In rarer cases, fibroids could even cause kidney failure.

Other symptoms from pressure include constipation, backaches, abdominal bloating, and discomfort during intercourse.

If you have large fibroids, you may also notice a pulling or stretching sensation. That's because your fibroids are doing just that. They are stretching the uterus and the abdomen as they grow, just as a pregnancy would. The difference is that if you were pregnant, your insides would get some relief after nine months, but you can suffer from fibroids for years.

Subserosal fibroids, myomas located on the outside of the uterus, are often responsible for pressure. Although they frequently don't extend into the uterine cavity, they do push out and may cause a swelling of the abdomen.

DISTORTION OF THE UTERUS

Every single day, somebody, somewhere, asks me the same question, "When are you due?" And I have to answer, "I'm not pregnant." It's embarrassing for them and for me. It not only affects the way I dress, it also affects my self-esteem. Who on God's green earth wants to look like they're expecting when they only have a huge fibroid to show for it? I just can't take it and I want this thing out.

My girlfriends keep telling me that I'm the lucky one because I don't get any pelvic pain, abnormal bleeding, or fatigue. They say they're really suffering. My doctor says, "If they don't bother you, you shouldn't bother them." I say, the condition I have is no picnic and I don't like knowing that they're growing inside of me. It's one thing to wear ma-

*ternity clothes when they serve as the means to a justifiable end. But in
my case, they've become a permanent fixture.*

—Arlene

The sistergirl above thinks she doesn't have any symptoms. But
Arlene's enlarged uterus, which causes folks to ask how far along she is
in her pregnancy, *is* a symptom. Fibroids are often the cause of a
woman's growing girth even though there may never have been a
proper diagnosis. I'm sure you had an "Aunt Lou" or "Cousin Thelma"
who seemed to look pregnant for years but never gave birth. Although
we all assumed our female family members were just gaining weight,
"often, these women had fibroids."[12] I thought my nana was just chubby
for years, but after talking to her about my female problems, I now realize she also suffered from fibroids. During the last few weeks of my fibroid saga, I could easily have been mistaken for being five months
pregnant. So I know firsthand that having an enlarged uterus can shrink
self-confidence tenfold and is nothing to take lightly.

Although we often wonder why the fibroid sufferer doesn't do something about her obvious condition, we need to understand that a dis-
torted abdomen is something that occurs over time and may be easy to
ignore. You don't wake up one day and find that you look pregnant. At
first, you may start to notice that your clothes are more snug than usual.
Unless your doctor has told you that you have fibroids, you may just assume that you're gaining a few pounds. But as your fibroids grow progressively larger with time, you'll also find that none of your strategies
to lose weight work. At first, as your uterus rises above the pelvic bone,
you'll have an extra pouch. But this small swelling will eventually re-
semble a pregnancy.

For me, I noticed that my abdomen got significantly larger right before my period. Once my period came, the size of my abdomen would
return to normal. The problem was that the normal size began to get
larger and larger, until it became terribly uncomfortable and painful.

CRAMPS

Sis, you may have been introduced to a lot of new information when
you discovered you had fibroids, but for most women having cramps is
old news. In fact it's so common among menstruating females that the
topic barely gets any attention. Cramps, technically known as dysmen-

orrhea, are the spasmic contractions that typically occur in your uterus during your period—although cramps can happen at other times in your cycle as well.

There are two types of cramps. Most women experience primary dysmenorrhea, which is defined as cramps that are associated with the onset of your period. Secondary dysmenorrhea is the onset of cramps after a woman has had pain-free periods. Women with primary dysmenorrhea may experience cramping so strong that it temporarily stops the supply of blood and oxygen to the uterus and this causes intense pain. According to Johanna Skilling, author of *Fibroids: The Complete Guide to Taking Charge of Your Physical, Emotional, and Sexual Well-Being,* "most women who have primary dysmenorrhea have had it most of their lives."

Women with secondary dysmenorrhea experience cramps later in life and it typically results from a medical condition such as fibroids, endometriosis, or pelvic inflammatory disease (PID). Fibroids, particularly intramural fibroids, may make cramping more severe because they prevent the uterus from contracting properly.

If you experience cramping, tell your physician when the condition developed so the proper diagnosis and treatment can be developed.

Take Notes

Do you experience cramping often?

_____

How long has this condition been occurring?

_____

At what times of the month do you experience cramping?

_____

On a scale of 1 to 10, with 10 being the most intense, how intense are your cramps?

_____

Are you able to perform your normal activities when you experience cramping?

_____

What do you take for relief?

_____

Do you exercise regularly?

_____

If yes, does cramping affect your ability to exercise?

PAIN

Whoa, if it's one thing I can tell you about, it's pain. When my fibroids were at their largest size, my back and legs would start to ache if I was standing for long periods of time. Then there were times I'd feel a sudden sharp pain in my side. My fibroids were starting to crowd my other organs and all of them were poking around for space. The discomfort was unreal at times and it didn't just occur during that time of the month—it was almost nonstop.

Another reason for pain from fibroids is red degeneration. That's when the fibroid gets so large it outgrows its blood supply and dies. This condition may come with intense pain, a low-grade fever of no more than 101 degrees, and some spotting or bleeding. For most women, the symptoms from degeneration lasts a couple of days, but be prepared, because some experience discomfort over several weeks. Fortunately, painkillers such as ibuprofen should provide relief.

Red degeneration can occur in any woman with fibroids, but it is more prevalent during pregnancy. If you think you may be experiencing red degeneration while you're pregnant, see your physician immediately for proper evaluation and treatment.

COMPRESSED BLOOD VESSELS

Large fibroids can put pressure on your blood vessels or nerves causing various issues such as varicose veins, hemorrhoids, numbness, swelling, or pain in the legs (sciatica).

PROBLEMS WITH PREGNANCY

A few months after I'd broken up with my boyfriend of five years, I came across some alarming information: he'd made another woman pregnant during the course of our relationship. Aside from feeling terribly deceived, a frightening thought crossed my mind: maybe I couldn't get pregnant. You see, my boyfriend and I were planning to marry, or at least that's what I thought, so we weren't as careful as we should have been and nothing happened—absolutely nothing. I was nearly thirty years old and my maternal instincts were in full swing. I wanted more than anything to conceive, but I never did. Miss Thing, however, hit the jackpot after a brief roll in the hay. I was crushed—to say the least. Aside from the other obvious concerns that anyone has when they find out that their mate has been cheating on them, I was also beginning to doubt my fertility. Was having fibroids preventing me from getting pregnant?

Experts say that fibroids are rarely the cause of a woman's infertility. Only a small proportion of fibroid sufferers (9 percent)[13] have infertility that is specifically due to this condition. But if that's the case, then why is it that whenever a woman is diagnosed with fibroids, her ability to have children is called into question or she is advised to become pregnant sooner rather than later? The answer, of course, depends on the personal views of the physician as well as the seriousness of the woman's condition. That said, research suggests that fibroids can impair a woman's ability to conceive or cause a miscarriage or premature labor. Although we'll look at how fibroids impact pregnancy in detail in Chapter 13, here are a few ways fibroids interfere with pregnancy (or proposed pregnancy):

Block and Stop

Fibroids can prevent you from becoming pregnant if they block your fallopian tubes or hinder the fertilized egg from settling into the uterus. But this is rare because it would mean that one or more fibroids are blocking both fallopian tubes. A woman can become pregnant as long as one fallopian tube is clear. Another way a fibroid can hinder a pregnancy is when a myoma located in the lower portion of the uterus during pregnancy blocks the cervix and forces doctors to perform a cesarean section. However, this condition is uncommon.

Protrusion and Intrusion

A submucosal fibroid can cause a miscarriage by thinning out the lining of your uterus and decreasing the growing embryo's blood supply. The good news is that a repeated miscarriage is unlikely because a new egg will probably attach in another location. Still, a fibroid that appears to be responsible for two or more miscarriages should be removed.

Chemical Crackdown

Fibroids may release a chemical called prostaglandin.[14] This hormone activates pain and may trigger contractions in your uterus. This is an unfriendly environment for a zygote that's trying to find a comfortable home in your womb.

There is scientific speculation that the presence of fibroids may also provoke a reaction from your immune system. Even though fibroids are mostly harmless and certainly not life-threatening, your body's natural defenses may become alarmed by the rapid cell division that is characteristic of these myomas. As a result, your body will attack the fibroid since it perceives it as an intruder. Unfortunately, your fertilized egg may be caught in the crossfire.

Grow Crazy

Since estrogen levels increase during pregnancy, you might think that your fibroids would start growing out of control after conception. Not so, say experts. A 1988 study of pregnant women with fibroids found that only 20 percent of them had fibroid growth while the fibroids in 80 percent of the women remained the same size. If you're one of the few women who do experience fibroid growth during pregnancy, you can expect your fibroid to return to its original size after delivery. And if you didn't have any problems with it before you got pregnant, you shouldn't expect any issues afterward.

Early Delivery

If you're a fibroid sufferer who has become pregnant, you can probably expect a normal, uneventful pregnancy. Although premature labor is sometimes associated with the presence of fibroids, most pregnant women don't have this problem. "For the majority of women with the tumors, the most that has been demonstrated is a tendency to deliver two to three weeks earlier than normal. This results in an insignificant degree of prematurity which poses little or no threat to the infant," according to the Fibroid Zone (www.fibroidzone.com), an online resource for fibroid sufferers. So if you're concerned about your fibroids affecting your pregnancy, don't fret.

DEPRESSION

When I found out my fibroids had progressed to a stage that re-quired a second surgery, I was thirty years old, single, with no children and no prospects. I was devastated and my doctors couldn't understand why I was so distraught. After all, "almost every Black woman you know has a fibroid."[15]

So why was I in tears at every doctor's visit? I was feeling desperate and terribly cheated. I had never considered in my wildest dreams that I might not ever have children. It wasn't even a passing thought. Women have children, that's what makes them women—or at least that's what I believed at the time. So when my doctor told me that I could be at risk for having a hysterectomy, I didn't think my life was worth living and I even considered suicide.

Sis, if having fibroids has got you singing the blues, know that you're not alone. Even if you're not suffering any symptoms from them, it's scary to find out that you've got uninvited guests in one of your most prized possessions. And if fibroids are causing you grief, that's all the more reason to be concerned.

But be concerned, girlfriend, not obsessed. I had to overcome my fears so that I could make some important decisions about my health. I implore you to do the same. There's really no room for panic, because it prevents you from properly evaluating the solutions that are available to you. Plus, excess anxiety can hinder your recovery. So what's the point?

Instead of going into worry mode, keep things in perspective and take everything with a grain of salt. Medicine is not an exact science, so your physician can only make educated guesses about your health based on past cases. Everyone is unique, and neither of you will know what the future holds until it actually arrives.

Also be aware that doctors must tell you the worse possible scenar-ios so that you can make an informed decision and so they can safe-guard themselves from a liability suit. And remember that your attitude will determine your approach. If you continue to expect positive re-sults, you'll be moved to select choices that will meet your expectations. More importantly, I hope you realize something that I didn't—at least not at first. No matter what the future holds, you are much more than a uterus. The essence of your womanhood is not between your legs, it's between your ears.

Give that some serious thought, girlfriend; then fill out the chart below. Your responses will help you clearly communicate your concerns to your physician. That's the first step toward a successful solution.

What's your problem?

Take this self-assessment quiz to determine whether your fibroids are affecting your body. If you have one or more of these symptoms, see your doctor for a more thorough examination.

	YES	NO
Irregular Menses		
Increased Menstrual Flow		
Pain or Bleeding with Sexual Intercourse		
Fatigue		
Paleness		
General Weakness		
Pressure on Bladder or Rectum		
Mucus-like Vaginal Discharge		

**Horus Global HealthNet.
The Difference of a Lifetime®**

Fibroid tumors in the uterus are excessive growth of cells in the walls of the uterus, usually nonmalignant.

3 What's Up Doc?

Establishing Clear Communication Between You and Your Physician

I don't remember having any symptoms of fibroids initially. What I remember is, when I was twenty-five or twenty-six, I went in for a Pap smear and my doctor told me that I had fibroids. I didn't know what that meant and he didn't try to help me understand. He had no bedside manner at all. He said, "You have a lot of them. They are very big and more than I have ever seen. You will never have children."

Having said that, he promptly left the room. I was in shock that he would speak that way and just started crying because I knew that I wanted children. He ended up leaving the practice. Physicians after that would say, "You have fibroids. Let's just wait and see what they do." No one ever tried to educate me. Everyone always said, "Wait and see." My cycle started getting heavy. I was given iron for anemia. I took birth control pills and Depo-Provera to regulate my cycle. The Depo-Provera made me depressed. I got frustrated, stopped taking all of the pills, and stopped going to doctors altogether.

—LaShawna McKinney, Age 34, Senior Secretary

By now, you've already been diagnosed with fibroids or you think you have them based on some of the symptoms you're experiencing. Whatever the case, a good physician is critical in the next stage of your treatment. The doctor you choose should have your best interests at heart and be willing to address your concerns in a unique, sensitive manner. No matter how many times he's treated fibroids, each case is different and he should try to develop a treatment based on your specific needs.

Now, sis, you may not even know that you have fibroids until your regular checkup at your gynecologist. That's okay, maybe you're not experiencing symptoms from fibroids or you're not very familiar with them. The important thing is that you find out whether you have fibroids, how big they are, and what your treatment options are as soon as possible. Above all, be sure that your doctor's diagnosis is accurate and complete.

Why? Most clinicians feel very comfortable diagnosing uterine fibroids after completing a pelvic examination. But it's important that caution be exercised here because although an enlarged or irregular uterus can be related to fibroids, it can also be caused by other conditions (see Chapter 11: Copycat). As one physician points out, "Because this diagnosis is such a common one encountered in the course of medical education as well as clinical practice, many practitioners in the past have been satisfied using only the pelvic examination without any other confirmatory evaluation. But all of us clinicians need to keep in mind that the initial diagnosis of uterine myomas really means that a given woman has a growth or mass in her pelvis. Based on our experience and training, we may believe that mass to be a fibroid. However, as you might imagine, this growth could be many other things as well. These include something as simple as a uterus which is minimally enlarged because of the woman having carried pregnancies in the past to something more serious such as a malignant tumor arising from any of the other structures which happen to occupy the pelvis."[1]

That said, only clear communication can ensure that you receive the best possible advice for your situation. This chapter will show you how to pick a physician that's right for you and help you maintain effective communication with the doctor you select. These essential elements are key to attaining the right treatment option to help you develop a healthier, happier YOU!

PICKING THE RIGHT DOCTOR

As I found increasing discomfort during my monthly menstrual, I sought medical advice. My doctor explained my options and impressed upon me that [my fibroids] were small and that I was not in danger nor did I have to alter my lifestyle or diet. I found this to be wrong.
—Janice Long, Age 40+, Teacher

A good physician is able to tune into the patient's feelings, consider the patient's background, and sense the patient's fears and anguish. It's a highly individual thing.
—Ifeanyi C. O. Obiakor, M.D., Brooklyn-based OB/GYN

Gosh, throughout my fibroid saga I must have gone through nearly fifteen physicians over the course of four years before I settled on Dr. Obiakor. He was highly recommended by my cousin, Debbie Slater, a gynecologic nurse practitioner for Cumberland Diagnostic and Treatment Center in Brooklyn. She told me the story of a woman she knew who had numerous large fibroids that had them removed by him and was now a healthy, happy mother. If he could do that for her, she believed he could do wonders for me too. But it really wasn't about what she believed; my fertility was at stake, and I was the one who had to be comfortable with my decision and the results. Even with her recommendation, if Dr. Obiakor hadn't measured up to my satisfaction, I would have switched again. What made him stand out from the rest?

For one thing, I appreciated his expertise. Despite the fact that I had my own health records from other physicians, he relied on his own findings to come up with a diagnosis. He also showed compassion. He listened to my sob story about my condition as well as my fears about being infertile because he realized that my mental health affected my physical health. He was also insightful and provided four specific reasons why he thought my fibroids should be removed: the large size, excessive bleeding, pain, and an indication that they were causing infertility. He then provided me with a printout telling me what fibroids were as well as the treatment options. In addition, Dr. Obiakor was honest. He was comfortable answering my questions (and I had lots of them) and clarified his expertise in the area of treating fibroids. As it turns out, he was one of the first physicians to perform a myolysis (see Chapter 5: Doctor's "Can Do" List) in my area; that was a procedure I'd had a few years earlier. That made me feel comfortable because I knew that he was familiar with a uterus that had been traumatized by that type of procedure, and he assured me that he knew what to expect. Finally, he didn't make any promises. As with any surgery, fibroid removal procedures have risks. He named some of them, such as excessive bleeding, which could lead to a blood transfusion, scarring, or an emergency hysterectomy. Now, his honesty was both good and bad. On the one hand, it made me a nervous wreck because I feared that I could wake up without a uterus and that would have meant disaster for me. On the other hand, it prepared me for the worst, and once I was able to deal with that, I could deal with anything.

But Dr. Obiakor was the practitioner I believed was right for me.

You've got to find a gynecologist that's right for you. I wanted a doctor who was going to help me maintain my uterus so that I could get pregnant—period. For me, preserving my fertility was paramount and I didn't give a hoot whether the physician was male or female, African American or a Martian. You may, however, prefer a female or want a black doctor, so you'll want to keep these preferences in mind as you conduct your search. It's all good as long as you're comfortable with your choice.

To pick a doctor that's right for you, gather your referrals, determine how you're going to pay for your services, find an office that has a convenient location as well as flexible office hours, and conduct a final assessment after you make your first visit. Review the following points:

GATHERING REFERRALS

"The way doctors select [their] doctors is to ask someone at the very best hospital in the area," says Dr. Susan H. Adelman, a pediatric surgeon and member of the board of trustees of the American Medical Association.[2] She suggests you take the same approach when seeking your gynecologist. At first, get suggestions from your general practitioner, friends, or family. Also, gain some insight by contacting the hospital that the doctor is affiliated with, because "hospitals conduct exhaustive background checks and have an intense screening process on physicians when they apply for hospital privileges and before they become a member of the medical staff," states Carolyn B. Lewis, chairman of the Board of Trustees of the American Medical Association.[3] Since a "credentialing application inquires about a physician's educational, personal and professional background, malpractice history, and any career gaps," these details may be available to you. See if you can get this information by talking with the patient care representative or one of the attending nurses.

There's also the web. You can scout certain web sites such as the American Medical Association *(www.ama-assn.org/)*, the American College of Obstetricians and Gynecologists *(www.acog.org/)*, or A Second Opinion Medical *(http://www.members.spree.com/angeleye)* to locate physicians in your area. In addition, take down the names and contact information of any physicians you come across in the media that specialize in the treatment of fibroids.

COVERING THE TAB

Next, check to see if any of the referrals you've received are included as participants in your health care plan. Start researching the ones within your health plan first.

Now, you may be thinking, "When it comes to my health, money is no object." Honey, you may not be able to put a price on your health, but insurance providers and doctors sure can. If you choose a physician that doesn't participate in your plan, you may have to pay as much as $250 or more per visit. But that's only the beginning. Any diagnostic tests that are required, which may range from a simple blood test to more extensive tests such as a pelvic ultrasound, MRI (magnetic resonance imaging), diagnostic hysteroscopy, or in extremely rare cases cancer screening tests, can start to add up considerably. And don't forget the costs of treatment. As an example, injections of Lupron, a medication that stops the production of estrogen and allows the fibroids to shrink temporarily, can run as much as $300 a shot or more, and at least three treatments are required. Even if you choose to do nothing, you'll still have to visit your physician every few months to ensure the growth of your fibroids hasn't accelerated. Make no mistake, treating your fibroids can be an expensive undertaking, and it's best that you let your health plan foot the bill.

Of course if you absolutely can't find someone in your plan, then a sister's got to do what a sister's got to do. But with the large selection of participating physicians in the various health insurance plans, there should be at least one that's right for you. And if you can't find one on your own, don't be afraid to ask a physician you like to recommend another gynecologist that accepts your health plan. Doctors understand that health care can be expensive and know that some patients must choose a participating physician for financial reasons. If the gynecologist doesn't want to recommend anyone else, then it's clear that your best interest isn't at heart and you should probably choose someone else anyway.

CONSIDERING CONVENIENCE

As with the purchase of a new home, when choosing a new physician you must consider location. If possible, try to find a gynecologist located near your home or office. Should you choose further treatment, you'll need to schedule a series of tests or examinations. If the physician is inconveniently located, then you'll need to take time off from work each time you have a doctor's appointment. Save your vacation time; you might need a few days to recover from surgery or you may require a break after this ordeal.

You should also look for a physician with convenient office hours. Now this can be a catch-22. Typically, highly skilled physicians are in high demand and it may take months for you to get an appointment with them. But you shouldn't believe the hype without investigating a physician's credentials. Some doctors are in high demand because they are good at what they do, but others insist on maintaining limited office hours so they can participate in other high-profile projects; in that case servicing their patients is not a priority for them.

There are also doctors who have poor time management skills. Regardless of the office hours they post, they can never seem to treat their patients in an efficient manner so they're always running behind schedule. They claim their tardiness is a result of their personalized care, but often it's because they fail to arrive at the office on time and lack proper scheduling practices. The gynecologist who first diagnosed my fibroids was also a practicing obstetrician. On several appointments, I waited hours for her to see me only to be told that she had to leave for an emergency, usually a delivery. Then there were times when I'd arrive at her office and find that all of her appointments had been cancelled. Her staff said that she couldn't help it, "in the baby business you can't plan for anything." I beg to differ. It was obvious that this OB/GYN didn't have a handle on her patient load, especially since she had no system in place to handle emergencies. I decided that this type of service wasn't good enough for me, despite her reputation. But maybe you feel differently. Only you can decide what's best for you.

MOVING FORWARD

Once you've gathered a selection of physicians that you're considering, let's say around three, start your research. As a start, surf over to the American Medical Association's web site *(www.ama-assn.org/)* to learn more about a gynecologist's qualifications. That web site provides basic professional information on virtually every licensed physician in the

United States. If all of the doctors on your list check out and seem equally qualified, go with your gut. At this point, you're only scheduling an initial visit, so if you find you're not comfortable with the physician you can still make a switch.

Next, call to schedule your appointment. When you call to make an appointment, pick a date that is between menstrual periods, because your doctor will probably want to do a Pap smear. It's best when you're not menstruating.[4] Also, avoid using vaginal creams or douching for at least seventy-two hours prior to your exam.[5] Pay close attention to the receptionist. Is she friendly? Does she seem knowledgeable about the office? Does she seem genuinely interested in your concerns? Even if she doesn't, you may still choose to forge ahead with an appointment, but you'll consider these factors in your overall assessment of your visit.

Now that you have a date for your visit, use the time in between to write down any questions or concerns that you have about your condition or the doctor's experience or qualifications. Just be aware that some physicians are more amenable than others to answering their patient's inquiries. If however, a physician does not seem open to your questions, that's a strong indication that you should take your business elsewhere. At the same time, your approach should be friendly and nonconfrontational. You're trying to get information, not to conduct an interrogation or earn a reputation of being a difficult patient. The most important consideration in choosing a physician is the testimony of the patients they have treated. Other considerations are:

1. Are there any malpractice suits against the gynecologist you're considering?

   This is probably not a good question to ask your doctor directly. Besides avoiding the risk of offending the physician, you want to receive this information from an independent source such as the state department of health; some states have recently established a physician's malpractice profile so that consumers can go to the web site to find out this information. Your state's department of health can provide you with this information or can tell you how to secure this information over the phone or online.

   One web site, A Second Opinion Medical Information Services (www.physicians-background.com), will investigate a doctor for a base fee of $135. Just be aware that this could be very costly if you're trying to research numerous physicians.

2. What medical school did the doctor graduate from, and where did he or she receive training?

Knowing their background can help you assess your comfort level before you meet them.

3. Is the gynecologist certified by a professional organization? If so, which one?

They should be a Fellow of the American College of Obstetricians and Gynecologists (F.A.C.O.G.). You can confirm membership on the organization's web site: www.acog.org. A subsidiary of ACOG is the American Board of OB/GYN (ABOG), the body responsible for certifying obstetricians and gynecologists. Board certification confirms that a professional body has said that the physician is competent to practice the profession of obstetrics and gynecology, but that is only one parameter of the assessment of a physician. There are outstanding clinicians who are not board certified, and there are very incompetent ones who are board certified.

Being non–board certified is not synonymous with being a poor clinician. There are reasons why physicians don't get board certified: (a) they are too busy to study to pass the exam so they don't take it at all; (b) they sit for the boards and fail them; (c) they are just out of training and have not reached the minimum of two years postresidency training requirement.

4. Is he or she a member of the American College of Obstetricians and Gynecologists, the American Medical Association (AMA), and the state medical society?

Membership in these organizations demonstrates that the physician is active and has an interest in the profession.

As said earlier your gynecologist should be board certified by a gynecologist specialty board such as the American Board of Obstetrics and Gynecology (ABOG) and have advanced training in areas such as advanced hysteroscopy, laparoscopy, and interventional radiology as well as the procedure that he recommends to you.

5. What hospital is the doctor affiliated with?

Are they affiliated with a good hospital? Good hospitals are based on patient satisfaction. In addition, good hospitals have state-of-the-art equipment and services as well as highly qualified, competent, and dedicated professionals. Most importantly, good hospitals have good nursing care. "Nursing care determines the quality of services," states Dr. Obiakor.

6. Does the doctor have office hours that work with your schedule?

You may not mind taking time off to see your doctor initially, but this could prove to be a big inconvenience over the long term and could cause problems for your employer. Plus, your paid time off will be particularly valuable should you decide to have surgery and need to rest up for a few days.

7. Is the office location easily accessible?

It would be great to have the best doctor in the business even if that physician resides in Japan. Most of us, however, can't afford and don't have the time to travel leaps and bounds to see a medical professional. Quality, of course, is paramount and you certainly shouldn't select a physician based only on their location. At the same time, you need to be realistic about whether you need a physician that practices near your home or office.

8. Is the receptionist friendly and accommodating?

Okay, it's time to find out whether she is as bad in person as she was on the telephone. Or was that friendly "may I help you" voice a fluke? You'll know whether your first impression was an accurate one based on how she treats you during a live meeting.

9. Is the office clean?

A clean office sends a strong message to patients: "We want to create an environment that's welcoming and inviting." That said, an untidy doctor's office communicates that the physician isn't very image conscious nor does he take the time to create an atmosphere that his patients will appreciate and enjoy. Neatness counts.

10. Do you feel comfortable in the environment?

Look at your surroundings. Assess whether you find them inviting and conducive to healing. Listen to the background noise and take a sniff; then determine whether you think the staff made a conscious effort to make their patients feel comfortable.

11. Did the staff appear friendly and approachable?

First impressions are lasting. If the receptionist doesn't give you a hearty "hello" when you arrive, that's not a good start. Also, look at how the staff relates to each other. Are they arguing or greeting one another with a smile? And keep your ears open. Tune in to the conversation and try to determine if the talk is appropriate for an office setting.

12. Did the staff seem knowledgeable?

There is certain basic information that the staff should know. For example, any member of the administrative staff should be well versed on the proper procedure for insurance plans. The staff should also know what services the physician offers, how long the practice has been in existence, and what hospital(s) the office is affiliated with.

13. Was the attending nurse competent?

Once you enter the examination room, your first encounter will be with the attending nurse. She'll take your blood pressure, weight, and other vitals. If you require a blood workup, she'll take blood too. How'd she do? You be the judge.

14. Was the physician open to questions?

By now you should have developed a list of questions to ask your physician before you entered the office. How did you find the response? If your physician wasn't open to questions, then that's probably not a good fit. You want to feel comfortable communicating with your doctor because you may be working together for quite some time.

15. How comfortable were you during the examination?

The examination should have been comfortable and pain-free. If it wasn't, then you should have expressed your discomfort to your physician and got an immediate response. Also, a good gynecologist leads you every step of the way through the examination. They tell you what they're doing and why. In addition, they invite you into their office for a private consultation where they share their findings and address any additional questions that you might have.

16. What is his experience?

New York–based OB/GYN Yvonne Thornton suggests you look for a doctor who has been practicing for at least ten to fifteen years. In addition, he should have treated several cases that are similar to the procedure that he recommends. However, it's hard to quantify the experience of the doctor in terms of number of cases they have done because you should be more concerned with their surgical skill than number of cases. "For example, a simple procedure such as drawing blood can vary by skill. Someone who has been doing it for fifty years may be no better than someone who has done it for six months because it is all based on skill level," states Dr. Barbara Gordon, a Brooklyn-based OB/GYN.

17. What were the results?

You should expect the overwhelming majority of cases that the doctor performed to have been successful—achieving results that are similar to those that you desire. Otherwise, find another practitioner. If there were any complications or fatalities, ask your doctor for the specifics surrounding the case. Also, find out what complications may arise with your case. Then ensure that the doctor has a strategy planned to avoid such difficulties.

18. Has anything unexpected occurred?

Find out what unexpected things can occur during the treatment process and hear what your physician suggests. Also examine whether any surprises occur during your visit. The treatment you receive should be reliable and consistent and continue to be up to your satisfaction during future visits.

19. Did the doctor give you a complete rundown of your options?

This guide should provide you with an overview of the options that are available for fibroid sufferers. However, your gynecologist should put the alternatives here and newer developments (assuming there are some) into context. In other words, they should let you know which options should work for you and why others will not. Again, the size and location of the fibroids, symptoms, and your feelings about whether or not you want to have children all affect which treatments are best for you.

20. Did you feel that the doctor treated you as an individual, or did you feel as if the visit were routine?

Sometimes doctors are so used to dealing with certain conditions that the treatment process becomes routine and they offer solutions out of habit rather than need. That's not cool because that physician starts to rely on the options that they're most comfortable with and not what's best. You can identify these practitioners because they try to make you feel as if your condition is no big deal and they push treatment options on you without considering your needs or feelings. Even though fibroids are extremely common, that doesn't mean they're normal, and any gynecologist who gives you that impression is less likely to provide you with a customized approach.

22. Do the doctor's goals coincide with your own?

If you want to have children and keep your uterus, your doctor should offer options that will help you do that. If he doesn't, then you should seek a second and even a third opinion. Even if you have no desire to have children, you should consider a hysterectomy only as a last resort because the removal of your uterus can have lifelong side effects (see Chapter 5: Doctor's "Can Do" List). In any case, you should be completely comfortable with the remedy that your doctor suggests.

23. Are you comfortable with your physician's bedside manner?

Although your physician's expertise is the most important factor, you still want a professional that's going to treat you with respect. You shouldn't feel intimidated, frightened, or ignored when you attempt to talk to him. In addition, your physician shouldn't try to make a final prognosis without confirmation from tests. So whether he says you have fibroids, anemia, polyps, or any other condition, he should be able to show you the results from specific tests as proof.

24. What factors contribute to your doctor's recommendation for treatment?

Again, some doctors provide all of their fibroids patients with the same remedy. Others may be influenced by the patient's insurance company. You want to ensure that the treatment prescribed for you is the best option for your specific situation. I suggest you heed the advice in the book *I Got Pregnant, You Can Too* (Underwood, 1998) by Katie Boland. She writes, "Doctors are only human. We need to remove them from their pedestals and lessen our dependence on them. Sometimes we know what's best, and that's why we deserve fifty percent of the vote. Seize it. A bad doctor won't give it to you but a good one will welcome the challenge. That's how you can tell them apart."

EXAMINATION EXPECTATION

Hey, remember your first visit to the GYN? I don't know about you, but mine was pretty traumatic. Five minutes into the examination I was at the peak of my anxiety and the attending nurse was patting the sweat from my forehead. That was more than thirteen years ago, but I remember it as if had just happened.

Even though I've probably been to the gynecologist a hundred times since then, I still feel a sense of anxiety before I arrive at Dr. Obiakor's office. But my anxiousness is largely diminished when I know what to expect, so that's why I think it's important that you try to imagine what's going to happen during your next visit:

Hurry Up and Wait

Unfortunately, many GYN offices have earned the reputation of being big on delays. There are a few reasons for this: latecomers delay the patients that come after them, the doctor arrives late, a patient has an unexpected emergency, or the office was overbooked to begin with. No matter what your expectations, you should start off this new doctor-patient relationship on the right foot by coming on time with the proper information. Promptness should start with you.

Review Your Notes

Doctors like patients who are informed about their bodies. They have a different respect for you when you come in prepared.
—Diantha Greenidge, Age 35, Accounting Manager

Since you'll probably have some time to kill, look over your notes. Have any additional questions cropped up since you started your initial list? Have you observed anything you like or dislike about the waiting area? Do you have any concerns about birth control, sexually transmitted diseases, vaginal discharge, itching, irregular periods, or pain? Are you having any issues with your relationship, intercourse, or any other part of your life? Write everything down so you can discuss them with your doctor; then review the responses when you get home.

Recall Your History

Girl, the nurse or your physician may ask you some private things during your visit. They may want to know how old you were when you had your first period, at what age you first had intercourse, when your last period was, how long it lasted, how many sexual partners you've had, whether you were ever diagnosed with an STD (sexually transmitted disease), whether you have ever been pregnant, and a whole host of other none-of-your-business inquiries. But don't worry, there's probably nothing you could say that would surprise them. Plus, the more information they have about you the better able they can help you. Everything you tell them is confidential—it's the law. Your secrets are safe with them.

Try on Some New Threads

Okay, so the robe isn't the sexy red number that you've got at home, but it'll do for this exam. The robe may be made out of cotton or paper. It may have snaps across the shoulder and close in the back. Or it may fit like a large jacket that you keep closed by tying it with a belt. It's designed for your comfort and to preserve your modesty, but it's functional and it enables the physician to properly examine you. The nurse may also provide you with a sheet to drape over your legs.

Relax and Release

It's exam time and your doctor needs your calmness and cooperation. As a first step, he may examine your breasts for lumps. At this point you will be either lying on your back on the exam table or standing up with one arm raised. The doctor will then open your gown to take a look at one of your breasts, then move his or her fingers over your breast in a circular motion. The physician will press lightly to attempt to feel lumps or anything unusual and will also gently squeeze the nipple to look for a discharge from your nipple or other distortions. He'll repeat the same procedure on the other breast. The process, which will only take a few minutes, should be pain-free, and you'll probably feel tenderness only near the time you're expected to menstruate. If you're experiencing any discomfort during this part of the exam or have any concerns, let your doctor know.

Next your doctor will perform a pelvic exam. As you lie flat on the table, you'll be asked to scoot your bottom all the way to the edge. Then put your feet in stirrups. This will provide your doctor with a clear view of your vagina. With a bright light, magnifying glass, speculum, and accompanying nurse, your doctor is ready to check you out. The speculum, which may feel cold at first, is inserted and expanded so your doctor can spread the walls of the vagina apart and look for abnormalities. This is also the point when he'll perform a pap test (or papanicolaou test), which detects cervical abnormalities, and a possible culture to check for gonorrhea and chlamydia. The pap is performed by inserting a small plastic spatula to collect cells from your cervix and upper vagina. These cells will be put on a slide or in a solution (thin prep) and sent to a lab to check for cervical cancer. You should have a pap test annually because the procedure can detect cervical abnormalities long before they become a danger to your health.[6] If you're sexually active, you should also be regularly tested for sexually transmitted diseases.

After your pap test, your physician will remove the speculum, and he'll insert two latex-covered fingers in your vagina to push the uterus up toward the abdomen wall as he pushes down on your abdomen with one hand. This allows him to feel the size and shape of your uterus and ovaries. At this point, he can detect whether certain conditions such as fibroids or a pregnancy are distorting the size or shape of the uterus.

Before a woman reaches menopause, each ovary is about the size of a walnut and can be felt on either side of the uterus during an examination, according to William H. Parker, M.D., author of *A Gynecologist's Second Opinion* (Plume/Penguin, $13.95). If the ovaries are abnormally large, this can indicate cysts, benign tumors, or in rare cases cancer. The fallopian tubes, which are soft and flexible, cannot be felt during the examination. However, tenderness around the tubes may suggest an infection. That area may also feel tender if you suffer from endometriosis or have scar tissue from previous surgery.

At the conclusion of your vaginal exam, your doctor will perform a rectal-vaginal exam, which consists of one finger in the rectum and one finger in the vagina. "This procedure will enable the doctor to do two things, feel masses posteriorly and check the stool for blood," states Dr. Barbara Gordon. "If you do find blood in the stool, then that's a sign that further testing is necessary. You really shouldn't have blood in your stool," she cautions.

Sometimes the gynecologist will perform the Stool Guaiarc test to assess the stool for blood. "You put a sample of the stool on this card and then you use a developer. If it changes color, then it means blood is present," she explains. "If it's positive, you want the person to go for further testing. It's a simple way to test for colon cancer and if you're a woman over 50 the test should be done on a yearly basis."

After your exam, your doctor will usually send you on your way to the receptionist so you can make your next six-month appointment and take care of your copayment. If your doctor has some concerns or wants to talk to you about his findings (such as fibroids), he'll either tell you as soon as the exam is over or invite you into his office for a private discussion. No matter what the doctor tells you, his findings will have to be confirmed by another test—so don't panic. Even if your doctor tells you that he's found a lump in your breast, for example, remember that 80 percent of these types of abnormalities are noncancerous. As far as your Pap test is concerned, the doctor's office probably won't receive the results back from the outside lab for at least two to three weeks, according to Richard W. Henderson, M.D., F.A.C.O.G., a Delaware-based obstetrician/gynecologist. "But that largely depends on the size of the lab," he explains. For the most part, you'll receive a phone call from your doctor only if there is an indication of some irregularity with the specimen. If you don't hear from them, that's a good sign.

Just remember, girlfriend, you have everything you need inside that pretty little head of yours to deal with any news the doctor delivers. So just relax, release, and be at peace.

THE BOTTOM LINE

Will practicing some of the suggestions in this chapter ensure that you'll choose the right physician? Absolutely not. There are no guarantees here. However, if you follow this advice you will minimize your chances of selecting a physician who doesn't have your best interest at heart. And that may make all the difference.

Fibroid Q&A

Don't leave your doctor's office without finding out the answers to these questions about your fibroids.

How many fibroids did you find?

How did you determine that I have fibroids? Your doctor's diagnosis should be based on a pelvic exam and ultrasound.

What size are they?

How large is my uterus?

Where are the fibroids located?

Are they likely to cause fertility problems?

How much have they grown since my last visit?

How often will we monitor them?

How often should I get a sonogram?

Do you believe the fibroids are the reasons for my symptoms?

What diagnostic tests have you performed to eliminate other causes for my symptoms?

What treatment options do you recommend? Why?

How do you feel about alternative treatments?

If surgery is suggested, ask:

Are there any medical alternatives for shrinking the fibroids or relieving the symptoms?

What type of surgery do you suggest?

Do you perform hysteroscopy in addition to an endometrial biopsy or the traditional D&C?

What are the risks if I don't have the operation?

Are you comfortable performing the surgery yourself?

How many of this type of procedure have you successfully performed?

What were the circumstances that caused complications with the procedure?

What is the estimated cost of the procedure?

Is it covered by my health insurance?

How long will I be in the hospital?

What is the expected recovery time (including time at home)?

What are the risks associated with the procedure?

What are the long- and short-term side effects of the procedure?

If the doctor specifically recommends a myomectomy, ask:

Are the fibroids likely to come back before menopause?

If they do, what are my alternatives if they come back?

What type of myomectomy do you expect to perform—abdominal, vaginal, or laparoscopic? (Opt for a surgeon who uses the least invasive procedure.)

If your doctor suggests a D&C for abnormal bleeding, ask:

How will this solve my fibroid problem?

What is the next step if the bleeding returns?

If the doctor suggests medical therapy, ask:

How does the medication work?

How likely is it to be effective?

What are the side effects?

How will this medication interact with other medications that I am taking, particularly birth control pills?

Will it have any impact on any of my medical conditions (high blood pressure, for example)?

How long does it take for the medication to take effect?

Are any of its side effects permanent?

How long will it be administered?

Can it be self-administered?

How much does it cost?

Is it covered under my medical coverage?

Will it affect my ability to become pregnant?

What will happen if I become pregnant while taking this medication?

If the doctor says "wait and see," you do nothing. This is conservative management. But you still need regular follow-up exams every six months.

Always get a second opinion from an independent physician who is unaffiliated with your physician when any treatment (especially surgery) is suggested.

Choosing the Right Physician—Points to Remember

- Be absolutely comfortable with the physician you select. Your choice is critical because this practitioner is making decisions that affect your life. You should be comfortable with the physician as well as his staff.

- Get a second opinion. Consult an independent physician who is unaffiliated with your physician when any treatment (especially surgery) is suggested.

- Don't rush into major surgery unless it's an emergency and confirmed by more than one physician. Try to preserve your uterus if you can.

- Choose a doctor that is a member of the American Association of Gynecologic Laparoscopists (AAGL, 13021 East Florence Avenue, Santa Fe Springs, CA 90670-4505; 800-554-AAGL).

Facts You Should Reveal to Your Doctor

Your complete medical history. Maintain a complete, accurate file of your medical background and keep it in a format that you can take with you to your office visit. "It is amazing how much [patients] forget," explains D.C.-based Dr. Tonja Gadsden in an *Ebony* article. "We need to know everything. . . . You can lie to your tax collector; you can lie to the mechanic. [But lying to your doctor] can be life threatening."

Your family history. Disclosing this information can help your doctor determine if you have a predisposition toward certain illnesses such as heart disease, diabetes, high blood pressure, and cancer.

Any use of prescription, natural, or illegal drugs. The information that you reveal will be kept in the strictest confidence. But telling your doctor what drugs you use will help him avoid prescribing medications that could be unsafe when used with other medications— that includes herbal remedies. St. Johns' wort, for example, can have negative reactions with prescription drugs.

Whether you feel overweight or out of shape. Perhaps your doctor can help you develop a healthy diet and exercise program. Plus symptoms such as fatigue could indicate other conditions. In any case, have an open discussion about your ideal weight, body mass index (BMI or percentage fat), and exercise habits.

Sexual habits. If you're having unprotected sex, be honest about it so your doctor can determine whether you have a sexually transmitted disease or if you're pregnant. "Untreated STDs never disappear and can prevent your chances of ever having children if they are not promptly treated," says Illinois-based Dr. Helen Davis Gardner in an *Ebony* article. "Many patients are afraid to bring those symptoms to light, but symptoms that are brought up early may save your life."

Your mental state. If you have the "blues," your physician is prepared to help you, so communicate any concerns you have about your physical and mental health. There are also remedies for emotional pain and discomfort, but you just have to let your practitioner know how you feel and be open for suggestions.

Source: "What Every Woman Should Tell Her Doctor," *Ebony*, March 2001.

WHAT IF MY INSURANCE CARRIER DENIES COVERAGE OF MY TREATMENT?

- Thoroughly reread your insurance handbook to confirm their judgment.
- Contact your insurance carrier and ask questions.
- File an appeal as specified by your human resources department or carrier.
- Contact your legislative representatives, get their contact information from the Patient Advocacy website (http://www.patient advocacy.org) or get a free copy of the U.S. Congress Handbook State Edition by the National Committee to Preserve Social Security and Medicare (800-966-1935).
- Appeal by contacting the medical insurance regulatory body for your state.

Get the contact information from the:

National Association of Insurance Commissioners
120 W. 12th Street, Suite 1100
Kansas City, MO 64105
816-842-3600
816-842-7175

4

Decisions, Decisions, Decisions

Choosing a Treatment That's Right for You

My decision to have a myomectomy was based on my family history. I didn't go through the typical symptoms like heavy bleeding or cramping, but after talking to my mother I just felt I'd have the same female problems as the other women in my family. My mother had a partial hysterectomy at age twenty-five, and three out of five of her sisters had hysterectomies as well. The youngest one of my aunts is only five years older than I am, and she ended up having a hysterectomy at thirty-six. She let her pain get to the point where the doctors couldn't save her organs, and now she'll never get a chance to bear children. I didn't want this to happen to me, so I decided to act on it sooner rather than later. I knew it was just something that needed to be done and I trusted in the grace of God for deliverance.

It's been four years since the surgery and I haven't had any problems. My last exam was in late June, and even though the fibroids came back I don't have any symptoms. Last time, I had five fibroids and one was huge. This time they're not as big and my doctor just wants us to monitor them. I'm just glad I took control of the situation.

—Peaches

So you've been diagnosed with fibroids and you're wondering what you should do? Join the club. Every fibroid sufferer has the same question when diagnosed: "What next?"

Your options largely depend on your fibroid symptoms and whether or not you want to have children. But your doctor may not tell you this because his experiences, expertise, training, and perceptions about what he thinks is best for you may taint his advice. That's why it's so important to pick a gynecologist that's right for you (see Chapter 3).

Bottom line, you have four basic options: surgery (hysterectomy, myolysis, myomectomy, or uterine artery embolization), medication, natural remedies, and the wait-and-see approach. Depending on the physician, a hysterectomy may be presented as your only option because of the size of your fibroids and your age. But you know better. Women with large fibroids, including this sister here, have had them removed and still managed to keep their uteruses. So if your doctor is pushing for a hysterectomy and you don't feel that's the right solution for you, seek a second or third opinion. And that goes for other treatment options as well; see as many physicians as you need until you're convinced that the advice you're receiving works for you.

Now remember, your doctor can only make his best guess as to how your fibroids have impacted the size and shape of your uterus after an examination—and a guess, even if it's by a doctor, is not a fact until proven. The way your doctor can verify his initial diagnosis is by having you take further tests. This will help you and your doctor gather additional information so you can make some decisions about your care. Here, we'll discuss the various tests that physicians use to get an accurate diagnosis and tell you what to expect and how you can prepare for these various procedures. In addition, this section will provide guidelines that will help you evaluate your treatment options by using the S.T.E.P. approach, a technique that forces you to look at the *seriousness* of your condition, consider how the condition impacts the *timing* of your desire to bear children, assess the *expertise* of the physician providing guidance, and determine how the alternatives presented to you fit with your own *preferences*.

TIME FOR TESTING

Complete Blood Count (CBC)

Unexpected bleeding, which later turned to excessive bleeding and heavy periods, was the symptom that sent me rushing to my GYN every few months. Not good. It turns out that I was severely anemic; that means there wasn't enough iron in my blood to properly transport oxygen to my heart. Anemia can cause tiredness, weakness, headaches, irritability, and paleness around the lower lids and hands. Now I understood why I always felt pooped. I also developed another symptom from anemia—an insatiable craving for ice, a condition I still have to this day. But it could have been worse; some people crave paint or dirt or experience a swollen tongue, heart palpitations, loss of appetite, fainting, and abdominal discomfort.

An average hemoglobin reading (indicating that there are enough molecules in the blood that carry oxygen) is about 12. My own hemoglobin results ranged from 7 to 10; this means I was anemic. Even with extra doses of iron pills, the excessive bleeding prevented me from ever reaching an optimal level. Regardless of where your results fall, keep track. Aside from the symptoms above, anemia can affect how well your body behaves during surgery. In addition, an extremely low reading of hemoglobin may warrant an immediate blood transfusion. If your doctor does tell you that you have an iron deficiency, ask him about iron supplements, limit your milk intake because it can interfere with iron absorption (you should aim to eliminate it from your diet if you have fibroids), and eat iron-rich foods such as beans, leafy green vegetables and liver (if you eat meat). But too much iron can be toxic, so take iron supplements only as prescribed.

Sonogram

After concluding that you have fibroids, your doctor will probably suggest that you get a sonogram so that he can determine their size, number, and location. Sonograms, also called ultrasounds or ultrasonography, use bouncing high-frequency sound waves to create an image of your uterus and ovaries on a computer monitor.

In the majority of cases, a sonogram will have to be performed by a radiologist in an outside laboratory. It will require a separate appointment that can be made by you or your doctor's office staff. Sonograms are also used to monitor the progress of unborn babies, so when you arrive at the office you'll probably be surrounded by expectant mothers. If you think this situation may be uncomfortable for you, take someone with you for support.

Maybe you'll be lucky during your visit, but I've always had at least a one-hour wait before seeing the radiologist. When you make an appointment, ask if the office typically runs on time. This information is important because you may be asked to fill your bladder—drink about eight glasses, or 64 ounces of water—for the procedure. If you drink the water too far in advance, you'll never be able to hold it until you see the radiologist. You should probably carry bottled water with you and drink it about thirty to forty minutes before you're called in.

You'll be asked to undress from the waist down. For a hassle-free visit, avoid excessive clothing, jewelry, and pantyhose. Instead, wear a pair of slacks, knee-highs, and comfortable shoes. After you disrobe, it'll be the same routine that went on at your GYN's office. You lie flat on the table with your feet up in stirrups. Next, your radiologist will rub blue lubricating jelly on your midsection for an abdominal sonogram. By this time, you'll probably be ready to blow since you flooded your bladder with H_2O earlier, so be prepared to feel uncomfortable. You may also notice that your body temperature has dropped in response to drinking all of that water in a short time frame, so you might feel chilly. The radiologist will run the probe over your lubricated skin and hit a series of buttons to get a better view of something he's spotted on the computer monitor. Although you'll be able to see the images flickering across the screen, they probably won't mean anything to you. I've had a series of sonograms at various facilities and I've found that the radiologists do not discuss the results and will simply suggest that you speak to your doctor for details if you have questions. One even told me that they couldn't read the results. Of course, that's not true; they just don't want to run the risk of misinforming you or even inappropriately alarming you. Still, you can pose questions to your radiologist and see if you get a response. Even if you do, it's best to confirm what you've heard with your physician.

Another type of sonogram procedure, endovaginal or transvaginal, requires that the technician place a probe, covered with a latex sheath, at the opening of your vagina. The technician can manipulate the probe to see areas inside of your uterus. There are different schools of thought as to whether an abdominal or vaginal sonogram provides better results, although the American College of Preventive Medicine says vaginal ultrasounds provide the greatest detail.[1] Still, others argue that fibroids located on the outside of the uterus would be missed without the aid of an abdominal sonogram. I had both types during my visits—you may too.

A written report will be sent to your gynecologist so he can discuss the results with you at your next visit. The write-up will provide details about your fibroids including their size in centimeters, where they are located, and how many exist. The report may also include other findings including the presence of polyps, cysts, or other irregularities. Although sonograms are the industry standard tool for diagnosing fibroids, the results aren't always accurate. There have been cases where a prolapsed uterus, prolapsed colon, or ballooned-out, impacted small intestine was misdiagnosed as a fibroid.[2]

A newer technique, a fluid sonography, is when your uterus is filled with saline solution so that the womb is expanded and the fibroids are more visual. Three-dimensional imaging is the next advancement in this technology. This will provide data on your uterine volume and a sharper image.

Magnetic Resonance Imaging (MRI)

An MRI is a noninvasive diagnostic tool that takes pictures of your insides by using large, powerful magnets that energize subatomic particles within your body.[3] Although an MRI can detect a wide range of health conditions, it can also be used to uncover gynecological disorders such as fibroids. But chances are you won't have an MRI, because the procedure is much more expensive than a sonogram and not necessarily more accurate. Still, if your physician has some unanswered questions after getting the results from your sonogram, he may suggest an MRI.

If that's the case, don't worry. MRIs are painless and may be somewhat familiar to you. You've probably seen one on a General Electric commercial or in some science fiction flick. You lie on a tray that slides into a large tube. When you're inside, you're completely surrounded, so you might feel claustrophobic. If you're the least bit concerned about this, let your doctor know so he can give you a sedative to help you relax, or maybe he'll arrange to slide you out for breaks. In addition, consider wearing a Walkman so you can distract yourself by listening to your favorite jams. You can also try meditating or visualizing yourself in a place you love. If you don't think you'll be nervous beforehand and find that you're uncomfortable during the process, just hit the panic button and the attending technician will come to the rescue.

Remember two things about MRIs. First, large machines require large magnets and that means a greater expense. To keep costs down, the tube will probably be small and narrow, so don't expect a lot of elbowroom. Also, once the magnets start operating you'll hear harsh noises. That's normal, so don't get startled. Just keep your cool and it will be over before you know it.

D&C

D&C, technically referred to as dilation and curettage, involves expanding the cervix and then scraping the lining of the uterus (endometrium) for diagnosis or treatment. Although this procedure was commonly used, it's now used less frequently because the same scraping of the lining of the uterus can now be done in the office using simpler, more comfortable means that don't require an operating room or general anesthesia. The newer technique is called an office endometrial biopsy. Still, some doctors perform a D&C to detect endometriosis, investigate undiagnosed vaginal bleeding, conduct an abortion during the first trimester of pregnancy, prevent infection or hemorrhaging following a miscarriage, and remove afterbirth membranes in cases where the mother didn't deliver them during labor.[4] A D&C also enables your physician to collect cells from the lining of your uterus so they can be further evaluated for cancer.

The traditional D&C procedure is performed in an operating room on an outpatient basis, so you'll need to complete the same forms that you would for any other surgery. A D&C may require general or local anesthetic or both, depending on your condition and whether the doctor finds a potential problem.

The first part of this procedure is the dilation or opening of your cervix.

The second component of a D&C is curettage, derived from the word *curette,* that's the suction instrument or looped knife used to scrape the lining of the uterus after you're dilated. The tissue that's extracted may or may not remedy conditions such as heavy or irregular bleeding. In any case, it will be sent to a lab for further evaluation. Be aware that you may experience some pain or cramping after the procedure if you're only under local anesthetic.

After a D&C, you may experience mild discomfort for one to two days and your uterus is going to be sensitive. It may take from four to six weeks for full recovery, but there are some things you can do to prevent further irritation. For one, avoid wearing panties made from any non-ventilating materials such as silk, polyester, or nylon. Instead, wear underpants with a cotton crotch. Also, no intercourse or foreplay that involves putting fingers, toes (can you imagine?), or anything else into your vagina during your recovery or at least until the spotting stops. In addition, switch from tampons to sanitary napkins for this time period as well.[5] And if your doctor puts you on antibiotics to prevent infection, be aware that this drug can reduce the effectiveness of the pill so you may need another form of contraception temporarily, but you shouldn't be having sex right now anyway, girlfriend—your body needs to heal.

Complications from this procedure are pretty rare, occurring in 3 percent of patients according to Johanna Skilling. The risks surrounding this procedure may include injury to the cervix, uterus, bladder, or bowel; infection (endometritis); and excessive bleeding. Call your doctor if your vaginal discharge has an odor or starts to increase, you experience vaginal swelling or abnormal bleeding, your pain does not respond to medication, you develop a fever, or you have additional unexplained symptoms.

Since a D&C is limited to the inside of the womb, it doesn't give the doctor any insight about fibroids that may be located within the uterine wall or on the outside of the uterine cavity. So D&Cs most often are coupled with another test or require a follow-up procedure. Also, if your doctor discovers a condition that requires a more extensive procedure as a remedy, he needs your permission to perform it, so talk to him about this possibility before the surgery.

But again, D&Cs are becoming less standard, so if your doctor suggests this diagnostic technique, find out why he didn't suggest a less invasive procedure such as a hysteroscopy, for example.

Hysteroscopy

Unlike a sonogram or MRI, this procedure can be performed right in your doctor's office but also in an outpatient facility or hospital. A narrow lighted telescopic device, sometimes accompanied by a camera attachment, is inserted into your vagina to view your cervix, uterus, and fallopian tubes. Certain conditions—abnormal bleeding, adhesions (Asherman's syndrome), polyps, pedunculated fibroids, blocked fallopian tubes, abnormal cell growth (endometrial hyperplasia), inherent malformations, and particular stages in cancer—can be diagnosed and treated through a hysteroscopy. In addition, this procedure allows your physician to take a small biopsy from your womb for further study.

With a hysteroscopy, your cervix is dilated and then the womb is expanded using carbon dioxide gas or fluid (normal saline). As the hysteroscope passes through the vagina and the cervix, images of the inside of your womb are projected onto a video monitor so that you and your doctor can spot abnormalities. Depending on his finding, your physician may use a variety of instruments for further exploration or to treat certain conditions. You may or may not receive local or general anesthesia for this procedure, but if you do, know that a shot in the cervix "can be more painful than the hysteroscopy itself," according to Dr. Fritz Wieser of the University Hospital of Vienna, Austria. So Dr. Wieser suggests a spray of lidocaine for numbing before injecting the cervix.[6]

As with all procedures, complications can arise. One issue that could occur from a hysteroscopy is a perforated uterus. If this were to happen, your uterus would heal quickly, but scarring from this injury could contribute to fertility problems. There is also a possibility that fluid could leak into your bloodstream. How? If your physician uses saline or another solution to expand your uterus for a better view, this fluid could leak into blood vessels in your uterus. An excess of this fluid in your bloodstream could cause seizures or fluid in your lungs (pulmonary edema). Other side effects of this procedure could be excessive bleeding, infection, or an allergic reaction to the substance used to expand the uterine cavity.

Laparoscopy

More pictures here. This time your doctor performs microsurgery on you by making small incisions through your navel so he can insert a tiny camera through the abdomen to look at the outside of your uterus, tubes and organs. This is why a laparoscopy is sometimes referred to as "Band-Aid" or "belly button" surgery.[7] As a first step, your doctor will insert a hollow needle through your abdomen to pump your uterus up with carbon dioxide (CO_2). The examination table will be angled so that the bowel and CO_2 will flow upward (toward your head). Next the laparoscope will be inserted through an abdominal incision so your doctor can get a closer look at the organs within the abdomen. At times, additional small incisions are made to accommodate other instruments. This procedure is more invasive but allows your physician to get a clearer picture of your uterus and surrounding pelvic area.

Expect to have this surgical procedure performed in a hospital, although it'll probably be on an outpatient basis. You'll require a local or general anesthetic, so talk to your doctor about his preferences and express your concerns. There are benefits and shortcomings to both.

Local anesthesia allows you to be alert during the procedure, so you can observe or ask questions. But you will also be aware of any complications that occur, and being awake during the procedure could make you more nervous. If you select general anesthesia, you'll be out like a light before you know it. Your recovery time, however, may be somewhat longer because you'll have to get over the effects of the anesthesia and the incision. Whatever the case, just be sure to let your doctor know if you have any allergies or have had any effects from anesthesia in the past.

As far as risks are concerned, you could suffer a puncture to a blood vessel and on rare occasions a perforation to your liver and bowel. Certain conditions such as being overweight, smoking, and heart or lung problems may increase your likelihood of complications. There are also medications such as diuretics, antiarrythmics, antihypertensives, and beta-adrenergic blockers that could contribute to difficulties as well.[8]

After you're released, you'll probably bounce back in a day or two. At first, you may feel bloated and find that your shoulders ache—that's from the pressure caused by the CO_2. You may also feel a little nauseated. As a tip, stay away from carbonated beverages or you'll feel even worse. Still, don't underestimate the seriousness of this procedure, and don't agree to a laparoscopy or any other surgery unless you ask lots of questions about the procedure and the recovery time. Again, if you're not comfortable with your doctor's responses or you're having second thoughts, get an independent assessment from another physician.

Hysterosalpingography

A hysterosalpingography, or HSG for short, is yet another picture-taking session that can be performed in a hospital or radiologist's office. Like a sonogram, an HSG can detect uterine abnormalities such as a developing tumor or a malformation you were born with. Plus, it can show your doctor whether your fibroids are blocking the fallopian tubes—and that's something a sonogram won't reveal.

How does an HSG work?

You know the drill. Disrobe from the waist down or change into a robe and lie flat with your feet in stirrups. Your doctor will insert a speculum into your vagina to spread the walls apart and allow for easier access. Next, he'll grasp your cervix with a hooklike instrument called a tenaculum. Finally, the dye injector is attached to your cervix and dye is slowly released while x-rays are taken. This will allow him to clearly identify any abnormalities that often show up as prominent distortions on the film.

During and after the procedure, you may experience cramping. Also, you may get an allergic reaction to the dye that causes nausea, dizziness, itching, hives, or low blood pressure.[9] If you feel too much discomfort, develop a fever (or other signs of an infection), or have symptoms for more than a day or so, call your doctor. He'll advise you to come in for further examination or can arrange for you to pick up a remedy at your local pharmacist.

Before you agree to have this procedure, there are a couple of things you should know:

- Test results are valid only for six months, since your fibroids could grow significantly larger after that time period.
- This test is dangerous to a growing fetus, so avoid it like the plague if you're pregnant.
- Schedule your HSG seven to ten days prior to your menstruation.
- The test should not be scheduled if you're having a period, have undiagnosed bleeding from your vagina, suffer from PID (pelvic inflammatory disease), or are allergic to x-ray dyes.
- Some complications from this procedure are injury to the uterus, infection, and an allergic reaction to the dye.

You could become more fertile following the procedure because a contrast agent, a solution that dissolves blockages, is injected inside your womb during the hysterosalpingography.

CANCER SCREENING TESTS

I've said it before but I'll say it again because I know people associate tumors with cancer, but fibroid tumors aren't cancerous. For the most part, fibroids aren't a health threat, but they can certainly be a nuisance. Still, if your fibroid is growing rapidly or enlarged, it may prevent a doctor from detecting other issues such as a tumor on an ovary. So if your doctor has any doubts about your fibroid being indeed a fibroid he may order more tests such as the following ones:

CT Scan

More pictures, honey. A CT (computed tomography) scan is another highly accurate x-ray used for internal close-ups. Its relevance in regard to gynecological use, however, is arguable since it doesn't appear to be any more accurate than a sonogram. Even if a growth is found, the radiologist can only indicate that "the suggestions of cancer may be present."[10] Your doctor would still need to perform more testing for a full confirmation.

Endometrial Biopsy

A biopsy (extraction of some of the lining in the womb) is performed if it's suspected that vaginal bleeding is due to cancer of the uterine lining (endometrial cancer) and not from fibroids.

CA-125

Once when I had a sonogram, the technician told me that my fibroids were so large that she couldn't see my right ovary. I freaked because I thought that it had disappeared into nothingness. Not so; it was exactly as she'd indicated. My large fibroid was keeping my ovary out of sight and it also prevented my doctor from examining it during my GYN exam. Since he knew he'd be getting a closer look at my ovaries and everything else during my upcoming myomectomy (although I was still walking a tightrope about whether I'd have it done or not), he wasn't too concerned. Your physician may feel differently if he can't examine your ovaries during a manual exam, so he might request a CA-125 to test for ovarian cancer.

Here's how it works: Your blood will be drawn from your arm and sent to a lab for evaluation just like any other blood test. Then the technicians will see if your blood sample contains a higher level of "biochemical tumor marker," which is an indication that cancer cells are present. The caveat here is that a false-positive result can be triggered by conditions other than cancer such as fibroids, pregnancy, endometriosis, recovery from surgery, and even menstruation. So a positive result still has to be confirmed by another test. And you thought it was time to panic?

Doppler Scan

In her book, Skilling says the Doppler scan was "one of the coolest" tests she's ever taken. It's a test that I skipped, so I can't echo her excitement. Doppler ultrasonography measures just how fast the blood flows through the arteries in your uterus as well as through the vessels that go to your fibroid. For the most part, cancerous growths draw blood at a faster rate than fibroids. What's intriguing about this test is that you can actually hear your blood through the probe that the technician inserts into your vagina. According to Skilling, "listening to your blood is like listening to the ocean only knowing all that power and energy is harnessed inside of you."

All of these tests can be dizzying, but now that you've been formerly introduced to each of these evaluation techniques you can have an intelligent conversation with your doctor about them. Remember to find out what a normal reading is and then write down your own reading next to it for comparison purposes. Always ask for a copy of your medical record including your test results. Then take these results along with you when you visit a new physician.

NEXT S.T.E.P.

It looks like it's time for surgery, especially if I want to have children later on. My doctor told me that if I got pregnant the fibroids would grow and there wouldn't be enough room for the baby to develop so the pregnancy would automatically abort itself. . . . Surgery is not my first choice but if changing my diet doesn't provide me with some results in three months I'm going back to my regular [traditional] doctor.

—Andrea Jameson, Age 39, Accountant

Okay, so you've been pricked, prodded, and pictured, but the question remains: "What next?" I suggest you use the S.T.E.P. approach to come up with a course of action—which may be none at all. Try the following technique:

Step One: Consider the Seriousness of Your Condition

If the results from your tests haven't revealed anything for you to be alarmed about, then you should probably just sit tight and see your physician for a follow-up exam in a few months. On the other hand, if results do show some cause for concern, take action. Just make sure that your response matches your condition. For example, don't rush into having a myomectomy (abdominal surgery to remove your fibroids) if you're experiencing some discomfort during your period—an aspirin might provide the relief you need. On the other hand, a hysterectomy is the recommended treatment for any type of uterine cancer according to experts.

Once you get the results of any test, ask your doctor to tell you what he suggests you do next and when you should get started. No matter how urgent the situation, take at least twenty-four hours to digest what you've heard and think about whether your doctor's advice makes sense to you. And remember it's better to be safe than sorry, girlfriend, so get a second opinion before you have any procedure.

Step Two: Know What Time It Is

If you want to have children, you need your uterus. Now, I know that should be pretty obvious to everyone, but when I hear women say that their doctors told them to get their uterus removed just as flippantly as your dentist would suggest you get a tooth pulled, I wonder if people know the real value of the uterus. Particularly since hysterectomies are even being suggested to women who are in their twenties! If you want to have children, keep your uterus—period.

Here's another point: even if you don't want children, you should still try to keep your uterus. If women didn't need their reproductive organs after childbearing, their uteruses, fallopian tubes, and ovaries would shrivel up and disappear. But that's not the case, so it's imperative that you hold on to these vital parts for as long as you can. Plus, there are some real side effects that can develop once you let them go, but we'll discuss that more in the next chapter.

On the other hand, if you've already had two myomectomies as well as other treatments and you don't want any children, then a hysterectomy may be necessary and increase your quality of life. Just remember, if you're nearing menopause, your fibroids will probably shrink on their own once your body stops producing estrogen, so you may be able to wait it out. And as we said earlier, a hysterectomy is essential if you have uterine cancer.

But a hysterectomy is just one of the many options that are available. If children are in your future, you can ask your physician about surgery, medication, or natural remedies. And if the fibroids are not too large, you can just wait and see. Just be aware that if your fibroids cause your uterus to grow as large as a twenty-week pregnancy (that's approximately five months and you'll be able to feel your uterus right beneath your belly button), you should take action so you aren't left with a hysterectomy as your only option. A full description of fibroid treatment options are in the next chapter.

So determine what time it is for you by asking yourself these questions:

1.   Do I want to have children?

As we said, a hysterectomy shouldn't be an option for you if you really truly want children. But also realize the longer you wait, the fewer options you'll have available to you because larger fibroids are less responsive to treatment.

If you do want children, do you plan to have them within the next twelve months? Experts say you should try to move your fibroid treatment, particularly surgical removal, as close as you can to the time when you want to have children because your fibroids may grow back and you'll be in the same boat all over again.

2.   Do I have a partner that feels the same way I do?

Now I know this seems like another no-brainer, but many of us women, and yes, I'll say many of us sistahs, are having trouble finding compassionate, compatible mates. We may have that guy who will take us out every once in a while but we know he'll never be a permanent fixture. Or there could be that old fling that's completely burned out but we continue to fan the flames anyhow. Take my advice, girl, don't get caught up in dead-end relationships because you think you can't do any better and are too tired to keep looking anyway. I've been there and done that myself a time or two and have found that it's better to hang loose than to hang out with a man that didn't have my best interest at heart. So save yourself some time, heartache, and in some cases money by either being with a man that totally adores you (yes, it's possible) or going solo. That said, if you want to have children but haven't pinpointed the father, you may consider delaying your surgical treatment for your fibroids until you've found Mr. Right, or you could have the surgery anyway and consider artificial insemination. Just know this procedure is no easy (or inexpensive) feat. I've flipped through pages of profiles trying to eyeball the perfect papa on paper and couldn't do it. I prefer the real thing and have decided to wait it out—at least for a little while.

Step Three: Connect with the Right Expert

At *Black Enterprise* magazine, we compiled a listing of leading African American physicians for the August 2001 issue by turning to distinguished medical professionals from the National Medical Association, Meharry Medical College, Drew University, Howard University Medical School, and Morehouse Medical College for advice. We asked all of the experts the same question: "If you or a member of your family had a serious medical condition which physician would you call?"

Use the same strategy when searching for a physician for yourself. Get recommendations from other physicians, specialists, medical organizations, friends, and family. (Refer back to Chapter 3: What's Up Doc? for additional guidance in this area.) But don't stop here; ensure that your physician's expertise matches your level of comfort. Consider how much experience your physician has with the various treatment options because people are creatures of habit and your doctor's recommendation may depend on his degree of interaction with the various treatment alternatives. If your doctor primarily treats fibroids with medication, for example, he'll probably make that suggestion to you. But don't take up the routine unless you think it will work for you. There's nothing wrong with finding a physician that has expertise in the treatment option that you want to explore.

To pinpoint the perfect professional ask yourself these questions:

- What remedy does my doctor suggest?
- How many patients has he treated using the remedy he suggested?
- What was his success rate?

- How many patients has he treated using the treatment option that I want to consider?
- Is that good enough for me?
- Can I get a reference? Some doctors may oblige, although most may have patient privacy concerns.

Step Four: Be Honest About Your Preference

So which treatment options are you most confident in? And is the option you prefer the most appropriate for your situation? Those questions have to be answered by you and your physician.

No matter what I suggest or what your doctor prescribes, you have the final say on your health. You may prefer one option over another based on your research or own experiences, and that option should be considered along with the others. My aunt, for example, recently underwent a hysterectomy. When I found out about her decision, I was upset, but then I realized she's at a different place than I am and she has her own preference. I'm in my early thirties, never been married with no children. She, on the other hand, is in her early forties and already has two children. Her concern was that she only wanted to have a surgery of this magnitude once and for all. She also felt that a hysterectomy would ensure that she'd never have to worry about uterine or ovarian cancer—she was right on that account. I still think a full-blown hysterectomy was an extreme move, but it really isn't about me. It's her body and her decision. The same is true for you.

WHAT DO YOUR TESTS MEAN?

"Treatment of fibroids is based on symptoms, symptoms, symptoms," states Dr. Obiakor. "There are women who have fibroids that are big as a nine-month pregnancy that are not bothered by them and they choose not to treat their fibroids. And that's okay. On the other hand, there are women who could have a fibroid the size of a pea but it causes excessive bleeding so we treat them. Symptoms are the true factors that determine treatment."

5

Doctor's "CanDo" List

Making an Assessment of Conventional Medicine's Offerings

My fibroids were discovered during a routine gynecological examination. After many years without symptoms, my periods suddenly stopped. Of course my first thoughts were pregnancy, but without evidence of other symptoms I doubted it. So, it was off to the doctor I went.

To my surprise he placed the blame on my fibroids. He also recommended a "partial" D&C as three months had passed since my last period. I underwent the procedure. I left the office spotting and had what I thought was a period. Thus the cycle began. But three months later we were at square one again. The doctor offered two options: another "partial" D&C along with taking hormones to shrink the size of the fibroids or a fibroidectomy—the surgical excision of the fibroids. I chose the former. I took the hormones even though they were quite expensive and not covered under my prescription drug plan. I cannot remember exactly how many cycles of hormones I took. But ultimately I had normal periods again and this ended my saga of the missing periods.

—Charlene Haswell-Jeanty, Age 40, Homemaker

Sis, there's good news and bad news when it comes to the treatment of fibroids. On the upside, there are more options for the treatment of fibroids than ever before. But these alternatives are still very limited in scope—particularly where large fibroids are concerned. Thus, a hysterectomy is still the second most prevalent surgical procedure for women; only cesarean sections are more common.

But hopefully you're choosing to act sooner rather than later so you'll have more options available to you. According to Dr. Grimes, a physician featured in *Health & Healing for African Americans: Straight*

Talk and Tips from More Than 150 Black Doctors and Our Top Health Concerns (Rodale, $29.95), "a fibroid that reaches the size of a 12-week pregnancy is the limit. If a fibroid grows beyond this size, the possible side effects include infertility or pregnancy complications, anemia, and interference with cancer screening." There's no disputing that big fibroids can cause big problems, and twelve weeks is about the size that they'll start causing problems. Still, there are women who've gone on to have beautiful babies and productive lives with large fibroids. Again, my fibroids were huge—well beyond the limit that Dr. Grimes describes. But why chance it? Explore your options early enough in the process so that extreme surgical procedures such as a hysterectomy aren't your only alternatives.

WHAT ARE YOUR OPTIONS?

"The choices regarding treatment of uterine fibroids are guided by the medical problems the fibroids are causing, your desire to have children, and your feelings and thoughts about surgery," writes William H. Parker, M.D., in his book *A Gynecologist's Second Opinion* (Plume, $13.95). "I think it is helpful for you to know all of the options available. At the time of the consultation, I usually begin with an overview of all the treatment options. Even if some of the treatments do not apply at the current time, your condition or symptoms may change," he explains. "If you understand the potential for future symptoms and problems, as well as the alternative means of treatment available, much of the mystery of fibroids will disappear. Once the unknown is discussed, some of your anxiety will diminish."

Dr. Deidre S. Maccannon of Michigan believes communication is key. "It's imperative that doctors spend time talking to patients and having their patients talk to them. Your doctor should be talking to you and educating you. Not just doing a sonogram," she insists. According to Maccannon, treatment options should be based on the size of the fibroid, its location, the patient's symptoms, and the patient's lifestyle needs. In addition, the solution should be comfortable for the patient and doctor performing the procedure. "My partners and I were shocked when people came in and said that other doctors said they should have hysterectomies when their fibroids are small and they only have one or two. . . . Having a fibroid doesn't mean you should drop everything and have major surgery. And you shouldn't trust someone just because they are an M.D.," cautions Maccannon.

Fortunately most women won't require any medical intervention at all, or limited treatment at most. "If your fibroids aren't causing you any problems and they aren't growing rapidly, the best therapy is watchful waiting."[1] However, if your fibroids are causing you problems such as pelvic pain, heavy bleeding, infertility, or any other symptoms (see Chapter 2: Sizing Up Your Symptoms), talk to your physician about further treatment. Here, we'll discuss the promises and perils of the wide range of available treatments, covering the wait-and-see approach, drug therapy, and surgery including myolysis, myomectomy, uterine artery embolization, and hysterectomy. If you're a candidate for surgery, refer to the "Surgery Q&A" sidebar for guidance. Also check out the "At-a-Glance Assessment Chart" for a list of all of the alternatives (including price ranges, success rates, and recovery periods) for easy comparisons. Finally, we'll close with advice on how you should approach your employer and provide you with a checklist so you can tackle this important issue with confidence.

JUST WAIT AND SEE

The vast majority of women with fibroids are unaware of them until their doctor feels them at the time of a routine exam, according to William H. Parker, M.D., author of *A Gynecologist's Second Opinion: The Questions and Answers You Need to Take Charge of Your Health* (Plume, $13.95). If your fibroids don't cause you any discomfort and aren't especially large (i.e., causing your uterus to enlarge to the size of a fourteen-week pregnancy or greater) then "your doctor will probably want to see you once or twice a year to monitor the fibroids' growth. These regular checkups (with occasional ultrasounds) can determine if there are uncommon or hidden problems, such as enlarged fibroids blocking the ureter."[2]

Sis, it's important that you keep your appointments when monitoring your fibroids, because growth patterns can change and could indicate a more serious condition. Although most fibroids remain stable, others can grow gradually over many years and then there are those that grow in spurts.[3] The only way to properly track their growth is by getting regular pelvic exams. "If you skip your follow-up appointments and the next time you come in, your fibroid is the size of a grapefruit, you may have missed the window of opportunity for managing the fibroid without surgery and may end up having a hysterectomy," according to Dr. Roberson, a featured physician in *Health & Healing for African Americans: Straight Talk and Tips from More Than 150 Black Doctors and Our Top Health Concerns.*

Just remember, in most cases, fibroids won't prevent you from getting pregnant or having a normal life. And fibroids are almost never life-threatening. Still, if the wait-and-see approach suggests more aggressive treatment, ask your physician to first consider one of the nonsurgical options discussed next.

NONSURGICAL ALTERNATIVES

There are a variety of medications, such as Lupron and Synarel, that you can use to treat the symptoms of fibroids, but there are no available drugs that can prevent or permanently shrink them.[4] Still, your physician may provide you with a prescription that can adequately diminish your symptoms so that you can at least postpone surgery or hold out for your fibroids to reduce on their own when you go through menopause. If surgery is inevitable, drug therapy may at least promote the reduction of fibroids so that your surgery will be less invasive and result in a faster recovery. If you're close to menopause, drug therapy can significantly reduce the amount of estrogen your body produces until your estrogen production shuts down on its own when you naturally enter menopause, causing your fibroids to shrink. The problem with this method is that menopause is as unpredictable as the onset of menstruation—nobody knows exactly when this condition will kick in because the process could take months or years before completion. That's not to say that drug treatment alternatives won't work. Consider these options:

Nonsteroidal Anti-inflammatory Drugs (NSAIDs)

Nonsteroidal anti-inflammatory drugs (NSAIDs) is just a fancier term for good old aspirin, girlfriend. Maybe aspirin or medications such as ibuprofen and naproxen can put a stop to any cramps or pain you may be experiencing from your fibroids. Acetaminophen, another pain reliever, may also reduce your estrogen level and that could slow the growth of your fibroids. Unfortunately, none of these drugs did a thing for me. I hope you have better luck.

The Pill

When I was first diagnosed with fibroids, I was put on birth control pills to stop my uncontrollable bleeding. First I was told to take one a day, then two, then three, but when I was up to five a day I finally said enough. The bleeding was not slowing down at all. And the birth control pills were making me crazy. It was hard enough to remember to take one daily, so I couldn't remember to take the rest of those pills, especially since they were all supposed to be taken at the same time each day—give me a break! Then one day my boyfriend pulled on some stubble while he was rubbing his hands across my face. I was growing a beard—can you imagine? Plus, my follow-up visits were even more horrifying because the fibroids were growing at an alarming rate. Birth control pills just didn't work for me. But that was my experience. Sometimes the pill can help your body control excessive bleeding and that may provide you with the relief you need. Just be aware that the pill can also make existing fibroids grow. So it's important that your doctor prescribe a low-estrogen pill.

GnRH-Based Drugs—Lupron and Synarel

Gonadotropin-releasing hormone (GnRH) is a hormone produced by the brain that regulates the menstrual cycle. But two GnRH-based drugs—Lupron and Synarel—temporarily shut down the menstrual cycle by turning off the ovaries' ability to produce estrogen and progesterone. And since fibroids need estrogen to grow, this reduction causes them to shrink. Turning off your period will also allow you to build up your iron if you're suffering from anemia as a result of having fibroids. This could prevent the need for a blood transfusion during surgery.

Both Lupron and Synarel are destroyed by fluids in the stomach, so they can't be taken as a pill. Lupron is administered in the form of an injection on a monthly basis. Synarel is used as a nasal spray twice a day. Both drugs are used over a period of three months. You can expect a 50 percent reduction in the size of your fibroids over this time period, but further reduction after the third month is highly uncommon. Also, shrinkage is temporary, so your fibroids will return to their original size after you stop the medication.

So what's the point? Again, these drugs are used to provide you with some relief until you can prepare your body for surgery or enter menopause. But since the exact time of menopause is unpredictable, the drugs may not provide you with the results you need.

One physician recommended Lupron prior to my first surgical procedure back in 1997. My fibroids shrank tremendously, but whether that was a good thing is questionable. Within three months of my surgery, the fibroids came back. Perhaps a few of the fibroids had shrunk so much that they were undetectable by the operating physician. But after I stopped using Lupron, the fibroids that were out of sight reappeared and reintroduced me to worse troubles than before.

And then there were the side effects. These drugs send your body into a temporary menopause and you feel everything that goes along with the condition. While I was taking Lupron, I suffered many of the same symptoms menopausal women experience. At night I would wake up in drenched pajamas from night sweats and would often throw off the covers in the dead of winter because I was suffering from hot flashes. Although I didn't use either of them, progesterone pills and the medication Bellergal can relieve hot flashes. However, progesterone impairs the effectiveness of GnRH-based drugs when administered during the first three months, and Bellergal may cause sleepiness. Users of Lupron or Synarel have also reported moderate vaginal bleeding for a week or two, vaginal dryness, painful intercourse, nasal irritation (specifically for Synarel users), and in rare instances headaches. The maximum benefit from these drugs is usually achieved over a three-month period, so surgery is scheduled shortly after that time period. Plus, you wouldn't want to use these drugs for the long term anyway because the use of these drugs for a period of six or more months could result in more serious side effects that may prevent your body from properly absorbing calcium—a condition that could lead to osteoporosis (thinning bones).[v]

Another shortcoming of these GnRH-based drugs is their high price tags, which could run about $300 a month over the course of treatment. Dr. Parker tries to help his Lupron users to split the cost of the treatments by getting his nurses to schedule appointments for two patients within a day of each other. Once a bottle of Lupron is opened, it remains active only for a twenty-four-hour period. Each patient uses half of the bottle and that's the dose required for treatment. "It takes a fair amount of time for our nurses to coordinate two women on the same schedule," he says. "But the savings for the patients are worth the effort."

Danocrine

Danocrine is another form of drug therapy. It's developed from the male hormone testosterone. Like GnRH-based medications, it stops ovulation and ceases menstruation; this puts an end to one of the most serious fibroid symptoms—abnormal bleeding. However, the side effects Danocrine causes can be unpleasant, to say the least. With the male hormone at work, you could experience weight gain, oily skin, bloating, pimples, moodiness, and facial hair growth. Given these types of side effects and the increased use of GnRH-based drugs, physicians like Dr. Parker don't recommend Danocrine as a treatment option. Can you blame them?

SURGICAL ALTERNATIVES

Sis, if you're experiencing uncontrollable heavy bleeding, if there's an indication that the fibroids are causing kidney damage, or if your doctor feels your rapidly growing fibroids are possibly other cancerous tumors (which is extremely rare), you require surgery. Infertility, excruciating pain (that doesn't respond to medication), and excessively large fibroids (greater than fourteen weeks) may also call for surgery. Depending on the circumstances, there are several alternatives. Each could impact your ability to become pregnant, which may or may not be a concern of yours, in very different ways.

Myolysis

Myolysis, also referred to as myoma coagulation, was introduced in the United States in the 1990s by Herbert A. Goldfarb, M.D., F.A.C.O.G., a New Jersey–based physician and author of *The No-Hysterectomy Option: Your Body—Your Choice* (Wiley, $15.95). The procedure is used to destroy a uterine fibroid by using a laser or special electrical needle to repeatedly pierce it until the blood vessels leading to the myoma have been damaged. This cuts off the fibroid's blood supply and causes it to shrink and die.

In *The Woman's Encyclopedia on Natural Healing* (Seven Stories, $19.95), Dr. Goldfarb details the procedure: "When we do this procedure, we literally undermine the tumor by destroying its blood supply. As we put needles around the fibroid, it turns blue, showing that the blood supply becomes interrupted. Fluid and blood go out, and the tumor shrinks. It becomes stringy tissue and just sits there, becoming very small, which eliminates the need for removal. The patient has no symptoms and can go about her life without the need for further surgery."

Although the cost of a myolysis may be similar to other procedures, this procedure can be more cost-effective in the long run, because it saves insurance providers money and enables patients to return to work sooner. "Patients come into the hospital in the morning, have the procedure done, and go home in the afternoon. . . . These patients go back to work within a week so there is very little cost in terms of disability," according to Goldfarb.

I first had a myolysis at age twenty-six. At the time I had the surgery, it was relatively new and it seemed like the best choice for me. Initially, my fibroids were too large for the procedure (women who undergo myolysis have fibroids of 10 centimeters or less—approximately six inches), but my doctor put me on Lupron and this caused my myomas to reduce significantly. As Goldfarb points out, the surgery and recuperation time is relatively short, particularly when you compare it to a surgical procedure like a myomectomy or hysterectomy. But this approach still has its drawbacks.

Although I was able to get on my feet in about five to seven days, it really took a few weeks before I was back to normal. Soreness lingered for some time. Also, the nearly nonexistent external marks from the incisions (which are three small marks that appear on the abdomen) are deceiving; the actual damage to the uterus can be extensive, since the procedure promotes scarring as a means to destroy the fibroid tissue. In addition, the available research on myolysis is scarce because the procedure is relatively new, requires extremely expensive equipment (more than $100,000), and is rarely performed in the United States. Thus, the long-term effects of this technique are only recently being uncovered—and that's caused concern for women who had the procedure performed in the early stages of its development.

In 1997, when I underwent the procedure, there was even less information available than there is now. So I was upset when I came across more recent reports indicating that this procedure should not be performed on women who plan to have children "because [myolysis] shrinks and denatures uterine tissue and thus weakens the muscle wall," writes Goldfarb. Now doctors share the view that this procedure could prevent pregnancy. But when I had the procedure, that had not been determined yet. As a result, I and other women are now finding out this alarming news—as if having fibroids weren't trouble enough. Also, since the fibroids are usually shrunk using GnRH before a myolysis is performed, there is a chance that your doctor may miss a few of your fibroids or new ones may develop. My fibroids came back with a vengeance in less than a year. Other women who had this procedure reported similar experiences. The lesson here is to ensure that any procedure that you choose has been widely tested before you undergo that type of surgery.

Cryomyolysis

Cryomyolysis, a newer procedure that could be considered a close cousin to myolysis (myoma coagulation), destroys fibroids by freezing them. By way of a laparoscopy, an instrument called a cryoprobe is inserted in the fibroid. Then supercold liquid nitrogen (-160 degrees Celsius) is added to produce the ice ball that damages the fibroid tissue.

Although this procedure has been approved by the Food and Drug Administration (FDA) it is not widely practiced in the United States, so the long-term effects of cryomyolysis are not known. According to Goldfarb, this technique is sometimes combined with endometrial ablation, an older procedure used to address excessive uterine bleeding.

Endometrial Ablation

Although endometrial ablation is sometimes touted as a treatment option for fibroids, that's really not the case. The procedure can be used to stop or diminish bleeding from the uterus. And that's important because fibroids and excessive bleeding are the prime reasons women have hysterectomies. Still, endometrial ablation has no effect on fibroids. In fact, it's recommended that you shouldn't undergo this procedure if you do have fibroids because the procedure addresses only the lining of the uterus and not the actual myomas. Plus, this procedure generally stops bleeding altogether, and that may prevent some women from receiving the one and only indication that uterine cancer may be present, particularly in older women. "If there is cancer of the uterus there is irregular bleeding and this prompts a woman to see the doctor," states Dr. Yvonne Thornton. "With [endometrial] ablation she has lost that early warning signal."

Here's how the procedure works: The surgeon destroys the lining of the uterus by burning it with electrical energy using a "paint-roller"-type instrument that's attached to a hysteroscope. The procedure could take as little as thirty minutes, requiring that you be under general anesthesia for only a short duration. So the risk of anesthesia complications, which is related to the length of time that the patient is under general anesthesia, is low. But there are other complications that could occur from this procedure such as a perforated uterus; injury to a blood vessel, bowel, or bladder; and the reoccurrence of excessive bleeding after the procedure. Expertise is paramount with endometrial ablation. "It should be performed in an operating room," advises Dr. Obiakor. "The procedure is very personnel intensive because it requires attention to fluids used for the surgery."

After an endometrial ablation, the ovaries continue to produce hormones, but no bleeding occurs because the lining of the uterus is no longer functional, and that also means the uterus can no longer sustain a pregnancy. The tricky thing is that you could still conceive in your fallopian tubes (also known as ectopic pregnancy), and this is a medical emergency that may require surgery. Although conception in the uterus would be extremely difficult, there's also the increased risk of spontaneous abortion, premature labor, or abnormal placement of the placenta. To avoid any of these conditions, you'll require birth control until you either enter menopause or opt for sterilization.

A spin-off of this type of surgery is uterine balloon therapy. With this type of endometrial ablation, a water balloon is inserted into the uterus and heated until the uterine lining is destroyed. But again, no matter how many interesting nicknames they come up with for endometrial ablation, it's still not a viable option for you if you have fibroids. You and your physician need to consider other surgical alternatives.

Uterine Artery Embolization (UAE)

> *I would definitely recommend that women don't suffer with fi-broids. Instead, they should speak with their doctors to see which pro-cedure is best for them. Then do some personal research and make their own decisions after being educated. . . . Uterine artery emboliza-tion was ideal for me because I did not want invasive surgery and I'm not going to have any more children.*
> —Leslie E. Royal, Age 34, Freelance Writer and Publicist

Another possibility, uterine artery embolization (UAE), is a techni-que that was first performed in France back in the late 1980s.[6] This pro-cedure cuts off the blood supply of fibroids and "kills the fibroids in the uterus, yet it spares the uterus itself," explains Dr. Francis L. Hutchins in a recently published article in *Essence* (August 2001, "Doctors We Love: Outstanding Black OB-GYNs Take Good Care of Sisters," 74). According to the article, the UAE procedure can reduce most fibroids by 50 to 95 percent. Currently, more than five thousand women have been treated with UAE worldwide, and experts say an overwhelming majority of UAE patients report complete relief of symptoms. There are some limitations, however. Some fibroids, particularly if they are older or scarred, may not respond to this procedure, so surgery may still be required. Still, many women can consider UAE as an alternative to a hysterectomy or myomectomy. That's why Hutchins, who is a professor of obstetrics and gynecology at Washington, D.C.'s Howard University, is on a mission to let women know about this option through his web site *(www.fibroidzone.com)* and publication *The Fibroid Book* (The Fibroid Center). "If people don't know their options they'll be victims of their ignorance," he insists.

So how does UAE work? First, an interventional radiologist (IR) in-serts a very thin catheter through the groin. Afterward he injects a spe-cial dye through the tube. The dye shows up on the x-ray machine so the IR can see how to manipulate the catheter during the procedure. Next he inserts tiny materials called polyvinyl alcohol (PVA) and waits for your blood flow to move the particles toward the arteries that feed the fibroids. Then the IR uses the catheter to guide any excess particles back through the other artery so they can be released. The idea is that once the blood supply is cut off, the fibroid will shrink, die, or soften to provide the patient with relief.

Expect to feel cramping after the procedure. Also, you may have a pink or brown discharge, as a result of your degenerating fibroid, which could last anywhere from a few days to a few months. Other side effects could be brought on by postembolization syndrome, where you'll develop menopausal symptoms such as hot flashes, moodiness, and cramping—a condition that could last from a few days to more than a month. There's also the possibility that your body could react the same way as the 1 to 2 percent of women that are thrown into menopause shortly after having a UAE procedure. Although there's no concrete explanation for this, one theory is that the PVA particles cause ovarian failure and that's why women who want children are discouraged from having this procedure. Further, an infection could also occur and a more serious one could result in the need for a hysterectomy.

The good news is that seven out of ten UAE patients do feel better, at least to some degree. And recovery time is significantly reduced; patients are usually released on the same day or spend one night in the hospital at most. The procedure should take about an hour, which is significantly shorter than a myomectomy or a hysterectomy. Plus, "the UAE procedure is no more expensive than a hysterectomy," asserts Hutchins. Still, there are a significant proportion of patients, particularly women with large fibroids (i.e., the uterus is larger than twenty weeks), that won't experience any significant improvements or none at all. If you're thinking about getting pregnant you should probably pass on this procedure because there has been limited research on how UAE affects fertility. Consider another option such as a myomectomy instead.

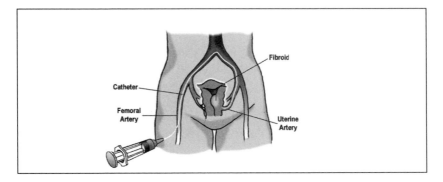

Uterine Artery Embolization

Myomectomy

> A myomectomy is the largest misconception of all and is not as easy as one would think. You lose more blood with a myomectomy than if you take the whole uterus out. Each fibroid has its own blood supply, and when you take them out they bleed. Plus, the woman's uterus looks like Swiss cheese when you're done with a myomectomy.
>
> We try our best to save her uterus if she doesn't have children. On the other hand, a myomectomy doesn't make sense when a woman has completed her family, has two or three children, and has large fibroids. I would not recommend that but we do it because many women believe that without a uterus they're not a woman so they fight very hard to keep it. If it's an organ that's causing you ill health, then one has to sit down and approach the problem in a very objective way that is in the best interest of the patient.
>
> The morbidity is much higher with a myomectomy than with a hysterectomy. You have to sew the defect up, and the large and small bowel oftentimes attach to the raw surface and women often have bowel obstructions after having a myomectomy. And after you go through all of that [the fibroids] can grow back again, to add insult to injury.
> —Yvonne S. Thornton, M.D., M.P.H., Board-certified OB/GYN

A myomectomy is a surgical procedure where the fibroids are removed and the uterus is left intact. This option, first performed ninety years ago,[7] is a godsend for women who still wish to have children since a hysterectomy was previously their only source of relief. Black women seem to be the biggest beneficiaries of this alternative because they get myomectomies at a higher rate than white or Hispanic women with fibroids, according to fibroid research conducted by the Duke University Evidence-Based Practice Center (EPC). Unfortunately the same study found a higher rate of hysterectomies among black women than other racial groups. In addition, black women were more likely to have hysterectomies and myomectomies at younger ages than other racial groups. But at any age, black women are more likely to have a myomectomy over a hysterectomy. Overall, hysterectomies are performed five times more frequently than myomectomies,[8] indicating that a significant proportion of women are unnecessarily losing their uteruses.

The school of thought is that if a woman doesn't plan to have children, she doesn't need her uterus. But if that were true, the uterus would just disappear after a woman reaches menopause and we know that's not the case. Regardless of your age or whether or not you plan to have children, make sure your doctor provides you with all of your options. And if he doesn't, find a practitioner who will.

The most invasive type of this method, an **abdominal myomectomy,** requires the surgeon to remove the fibroids by laparotomy (making a four- to six-inch incision through the abdomen) while you're under general anesthesia. Generally, doctors favor abdominal myomectomies over other techniques because the procedure is more widely used than the others, provides the largest field of vision that may make previously undetected fibroids apparent, and enables the surgeon to ensure that all blood vessels have been properly sealed as well as resolve any other problems that may have resulted from the surgery before closing up.

With an abdominal myomectomy, the doctor enters the pelvic area through an incision made through the abdomen. Then the bladder and intestines are manipulated so the doctor can see inside the uterus. Once it's determined how many fibroids are present, their position and size, the doctor then injects the uterus with Pitressin, a fluid that prevents excessive bleeding during surgery. Next the fibroids are cut from the uterine muscle and the uterus is repaired. This surgery takes about one to two hours depending on specifics surrounding the fibroids that need to be removed.

But the time you spend in surgery is small stuff compared to your recovery period. The intestines, which were handled and exposed during the surgery, could take a few days to operate normally again. When you wake up, you can expect to experience pain and soreness from the incision. The good news is that you'll be able to relieve your discomfort yourself because you'll be hooked up to a morphine tap that will pump you with pain reliever when you press a button. Don't worry about becoming addicted, the machine is set so that only small doses are released over certain periods of time. Plus, the nurse monitors the machine regularly. You'll also be hooked up to an intravenous line and a catheter (a hollow tube that's inserted into your urethra to collect urine), so expect to be on bed rest for the first night. You'll probably be in the hospital from three to four days. Before you leave, your attending physicians may ensure that you pass gas, have a bowel movement, and walk around (within the hospital, of course). Laughing, coughing, and sitting up will be difficult at first but you'll live. And if all goes well, you'll be fibroid-free—possibly forever.

Ideally, your physician would have entered your abdomen through a horizontal incision that would be made right below your pubic hairline so that the scar would barely be visible after it heals. However, if your fibroids are large, as in my case, the incision would be made vertically from the navel to the pubic bone. Unfortunately most doctors won't know which incision they're going to make until you're under anesthesia and they can examine your abdomen when you're relaxed. Regardless of what type of incision you require, don't sweat the scar, because I can almost guarantee that it's not nearly as horrid as the one I have on my belly. It's about as wide as a large, long pickle because of my skin keloids (we'll talk about that later). But I'm just extremely happy that I didn't have to have a hysterectomy (in rare instances, a complication during a myomectomy can result in an emergency hysterectomy) and that I can still have children. I figure I can't swim anyhow, so I rarely wear a bathing suit and don't mind opting for a one-piece on the few occasions when I do hit the beach. And since anyone who actually sees the scar from my myomectomy is someone that's supposed to be in that vicinity, say a doctor or my future hubby, I'm sure a big old ugly keloid will be the least of their concerns.

A **laparoscopic myomectomy,** developed in the 1980s, is another alternative. The surgeon inserts a laparoscope (small telescope) through an incision made through the navel so they can get an inside view of the abdominal cavity and the uterus. Then additional instruments such as scissors, a laser, or retractors are passed through the small incisions that are made below the bikini line to make cuts, clip, or repair. To remove the fibroid from the abdominal cavity, it's cut into tiny pieces (morcellation) and taken out through the tiny incisions. Depending on how many fibroids need to be removed, this technique can be time consuming, taking anywhere from one to three hours. It also requires a lot of eye–hand coordination since the surgeon is relying on a video monitor for direction.

There are both favorable and disapproving reviews of the laparoscopic myomectomy technique. On the upside, the procedure is usually performed as outpatient surgery under general anesthesia, so patients can leave the hospital the same day. Recovery is fast because the incisions are small and there is minimal interference with the intestine or other organs. Women undergoing this type of procedure can typically resume normal activities, including work and exercise, after two weeks.

Whether a laparoscopic myomectomy should be performed on a

woman who desires children is controversial. Some surgeons claim that the uterus is not repaired securely enough to safely carry a developing baby or withstand the stress of labor after this type of surgery. Physicians often recommend that women who've undergone a laparoscopic myomectomy or "full thickness myomectomy" give birth by cesarean section. Dr. Obiakor strongly recommended that I have a cesarean if I ever became pregnant because I had a "full thickness myomectomy," which means that the incision on my uterus went from the top of the uterus down to the cavity of the uterus. As a result, there is a risk that if the uterus goes through labor it may split open along that incision during contractions. A cesarean is fine with me because I want to do whatever it takes to have a healthy baby.

Still, there is no real evidence, only theory, that laparoscopic myomectomy is any worse on a pregnancy than an abdominal myomectomy. So you may still be able to have a normal delivery with either technique. There's still the issue of overuse when it comes to laparoscopic procedures. According to Dr. Parker's book, "small fibroids that are seen during laparoscopy are removed when this may not be neces-

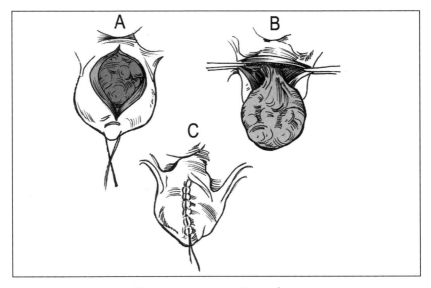

The Myomectomy Procedure

sary. . . . As with all surgery, laparoscopic myomectomy should be performed only if appropriate indications exist." Talk to your physician about any concerns that you have and ensure that your surgeon is highly trained and experienced in laparoscopic myomectomies. In addition, ask exactly how many times he's performed the procedure and what were the results. Also, have your doctor tell you about any complications he's experienced as well as any issues he believes that could become challenges during your surgery.

Just remember to take an honest assessment of your options and consider all of the shortcomings, cautions Richard W. Henderson, M.D., F.A.C.O.G., a Delaware-based obstetrician/gynecologist. "You may have [the fibroids] removed or destroyed. But as long as the uterus is in place, there is a chance that the fibroids will come back."

Hysterectomy

> They had to take out both of my ovaries and my uterus. I asked for it because I was 42 years old and I'd had all my children. It was a blessing because I didn't have to go through the change of life. All of this stuff that people have to take, I never went through that. I've never taken a hormone in my life. I was feeling good ever since that [hysterectomy] happened. I didn't have any symptoms of menopause and I could beat any of those women on the nursing ward working. I didn't have any hot flashes, nervousness, or nothing else.
>
> —Adele Brown-Anderson, Age 76
> Minister and Retired Cosmetologist and Nurse

A hysterectomy, which requires a doctor to remove your uterus, is the most drastic fibroid treatment. Historically, black women have hysterectomies at a significantly higher rate than white women and are also more likely to suffer complications from the procedure than their white counterparts. Researchers reported that of the 409 black women who had hysterectomies for noncancerous conditions, 89 percent had fibroids. At the same time, of the 836 white women who had hysterectomies for noncancerous conditions, 59 percent had fibroids.[9] Black women also had a 40 percent greater risk of hemorrhaging or developing an infection as a result of a hysterectomy and typically underwent the procedure at a younger age than the white patients (forty-two versus forty-six years of age). In addition, black women were more likely than white to have an abdominal hysterectomy (the most invasive procedure) than a vaginal hysterectomy (the least invasive procedure). Perhaps this could be partially explained by the size of the patients' fibroids. For black patients, their average uterine weight was 421 grams, while the average uterine weight for white patients was 319 grams. There is still some speculation that black women generally don't seek treatment early enough to avoid a hysterectomy and aren't given the full scope of options even when they do. And then there are black women who believe (or have been convinced) that a hysterectomy is the best treatment.

After all, once the procedure has been completed, your periods are gone, finito, caput. Plus, your ability to have children will be a thing of the past. For some women, that's a blessing. Others suffer devastation. Thoroughly examine your feelings before you move forward with a hysterectomy, and if you still choose to have one you'll be in a pleasant state of mind during your recovery.

There are various types of hysterectomies including a supracervical or subtotal, total abdominal, vaginal, or laparoscopically assisted vaginal hysterectomy.

A **supracervical hysterectomy** is when the doctor removes the top part of the uterus leaving the cervix intact. This type of hysterectomy is usually the least invasive because the top portion of the uterus is removed by laparoscopy. For the most part, pain and complications are at a minimum when this type of hysterectomy is performed. And since the cervix remains attached to the vagina and its ligaments, your sexual sensations should still kick in.

Should you decide to have a **total hysterectomy,** your uterus and cervix would be removed, but you'd keep both ovaries as well as your fallopian tubes. As long as your ovaries are in place, they'll produce the hormones you need to avoid osteoporosis and other illnesses. Like a myomectomy, the surgery can be performed through the vagina, abdomen (TAH, or total abdominal hysterectomy), or laparoscopically.

Vaginal hysterectomies are the simplest. There are no external or internal scars, and this makes recovery time much shorter than for an abdominal hysterectomy. The uterus shouldn't be larger than twelve to fourteen weeks in size, although some doctors say they can remove a uterus that's twenty weeks in size. The other caveat is that since vaginal hysterectomies are considered relatively hassle-free, they may be unnecessarily recommended. In the book, *The No-Hysterectomy Option: Your Body—Your Choice* (Wiley, $15.95), Dr. Herbert Goldfarb cautions against choosing hysterectomies in haste: "The thirty-minute vaginal hysterectomies that doctors boast of performing are often procedures that don't have to be done in the first place!"[10] A **laparoscopically assisted vaginal hysterectomy (LAVH)** is another type of vaginal hysterectomy. LAVH could help your doctor tackle larger fibroids without performing abdominal surgery or at least make the uterus small enough so that an abdominal surgery is less complicated. Opting for an LAVH allows the surgeon to check for adhesions or other issues that a prior surgery may have left behind before the uterus is removed vaginally. This could mean less pain and easier recovery for you.

An abdominal surgery, however, enables the surgeon to get a clear view of the internal organs. Its use depends on the physician's comfort level. If they've been primarily trained using abdominal surgery then that will be their preference. But abdominal surgery is also the most invasive and has the longest recovery time. You can expect to stay in the hospital for three to five days and your total recovery may take four to six weeks.

Surgery Q&A

1. Are you board certified in obstetrics and gynecology?

   Although there are good surgeons who are not board certified, certification does indicate that the physician has at least met some standard of competence. If you see F.A.C.O.G. (Fellow of the American College of Obstetricians and Gynecologists) after the doctor's name, that indicates board certification.

   ---

2. What proportion of your patients have fibroids?

   You should choose a physician who deals routinely with fibroid issues.

   ---

3. Do you perform laparoscopic myomectomies?

   A surgeon who routinely performs this type of surgery should be prepared to offer a full range of options for surgically treating fibroids.

   ---

4. How many laparoscopic myomectomies have you performed?

Laparoscopic myomectomies are the most difficult laparoscopic procedure that a gynecologic surgeon can perform and require extensive experience and training. The chance of complications is reduced if your surgeon has performed a substantial number of these procedures.

5. How many laparoscopic myomectomies do you perform annually?

A surgeon that doesn't perform a significant number of laparoscopic myomectomies isn't likely to offer this as an option for the treatment of fibroids. You should expect that your gynecologist to have performed at least eight to ten a year. Otherwise switch to a more experienced surgeon.

6. Where do you perform laparoscopic myomectomies?

The best place is a full-service hospital because your surgeon will have immediate access to special equipment, specialized personnel, lab facilities, and expertise in case of a complication. There are surgeons, however, who do perform myomectomies or hysterectomies in a freestanding ambulatory surgery unit. Just be aware that if a complication arises, your surgeon could lose precious time transporting you from that facility to a hospital.

7. Do you use GnRH drugs to shrink fibroids prior to surgery?

A physician should be experienced with the use of GnRH drugs in the shrinkage of fibroids and their ability to reduce bleeding during surgery. There are gynecologists, however, who don't support the use of these drugs because they change the consistency of fibroids and make them more difficult to remove. Find out your physician's school of thought and then decide if the approach works for you.

8. What complications have you encountered with laparoscopic myomectomies?

Risks with laparoscopic myomectomies are minimal, particularly in young, healthy women, but if you have certain conditions, the threat of complications can be increased. For example, if you've had previous abdominal surgeries, especially if the procedure involved the bowel or pelvic area, you may have scarring that could obstruct the surgeon's view and make the surgery more difficult. Infections, tumors, and obesity may also contribute to difficulties. Certain injuries resulting from the surgery, particularly from the incision-making sharp-pointed piercing instrument called the trocar, can include damage to a blood vessel, a bowel, or the bladder. Complications can also occur after surgery. Call your physician if you develop swelling, extreme abdominal pain, vomiting, a fever, redness, or drainage from the incision. Your physician should regularly discuss these complications as well as others.

9. How do you prevent excessive bleeding during surgery?

Nelson H. Stringer, M.D., author of *Uterine Fibroids: What Every Woman Needs to Know*, injects a solution of vasopressin (Pitressin) into the uterus during surgery. This causes blood vessels to shrink and reduces the amount of blood loss during traditional and laparoscopic surgery. The use of a harmonic scalpel during surgery also significantly reduces blood loss. Find out if your doctor takes any precautions to prevent blood loss during surgery, then research the viability of his suggestions with an independent source.

10. How many of your patients have required a blood transfusion over the last five years?

Experienced surgeons should be able to perform most myomectomies without blood transfusions.

11. Do you use and recommend autologous blood donation?

Remember, your surgeon should be able to perform a myomectomy without a blood transfusion. However, as an extra precaution you may want to make an autologous blood donation. That's when you bank your own blood so that it's accessible for a major upcoming surgery. To do this, "you must have a hemoglobin level of at least 11 grams or a hematocrit level of at least 34%," writes Nelson. You'll need to donate at least two units of blood, which can be stored for only thirty-five to forty-five days and must be used no less than seventy-two hours after it was collected—otherwise you'd be too weak to have surgery. If your bleeding is excessive and requires more than two units of blood, your surgeon would then need additional units of homologous blood (donated by others from the blood bank). The use of your own blood reduces your risk of contracting AIDS (which is between 1 in 400,000 and 1 in a million). And no matter which blood you use, you still run the risk of the most common complication, clerical error, where the blood bank mistakenly provides a patient with the wrong blood units. Still, using your own blood is best. Nelson says, "Autologous blood donation is ideal for elective gynecological surgeries such as myomectomy and hysterectomy, because most patients are relatively young and otherwise healthy, and a delay of 3 to 4 weeks from the time the blood is donated is not critical." Find out your physician's views on this procedure.

12. Do you use the harmonic scalpel?

The harmonic scalpel is a new instrument used in laparoscopic surgery and is very effective for the laparoscopic removal of fibroids. It's also safer than other instruments because it cuts tissue and seals blood vessels by using blade vibrations and ultrasonic waves rather than electrical current or laser energy. This results in less bleeding. Nelson suggests that you find someone who is experienced in using the harmonic scalpel if you're going to have a laparoscopic myomectomy.

13. Do you use the endo stitch?

Nelson strongly recommends the endo stitch for uterine closure following a laparoscopic myomectomy. This surgical sewing machine reduces repair time by an hour; thus the overall cost of the surgical procedure is diminished.

14. Have any of your patients died as a result of complications from a myomectomy?

The complications from a traditional myomectomy are similar to those of any other surgical procedure including hemorrhage, small intestine problems, infection, and postoperative blood clots in the legs. Deaths from myomectomies can occur because of excessive blood loss.

15. Have any of your patients died as a result of complications from a laparoscopic surgery?

Death as a result of a laparoscopic myomectomy is nearly nonexistent. If your surgeon reveals that even one of his patients died following this procedure, you should get additional details and seek a second opinion.

Source: Nelson H. Stringer, M.D., *Uterine Fibroids: What Every Woman Needs to Know.*

SO WHAT'S A SISTAH TO DO?

Chapter 4 offered the S.T.E.P. approach as a method for choosing the right treatment option. But you should also keep some facts in mind while you make your decision. For example, African American women are 25 percent more likely to have a hysterectomy than their white counterparts, according to research by the state of Maryland.[11] The same study also reports that African American women who receive hysterectomies are more likely to suffer complications and have a longer hospital stay. What was most alarming is that African American women were three times more likely to die from a hysterectomy than their white counterparts.[12] Needless to say, choosing to get a hysterectomy is serious business, particularly since it may also be unnecessary.

I find the thought of having a hysterectomy absolutely terrifying, but I guess you know that by now. So many of us sisters are told we need a hysterectomy when what we really need is further study. Just the other day, I was talking to another one of my aunts, who is on the brink of having a hysterectomy. Her periods wreak havoc every month and as far as she's decided it's time to get rid of her troubling uterus.

Maybe having a hysterectomy is the best choice for her. After all, she has three children and is over forty, and she's cool with the idea. But there are many women who don't have the same set of circumstances and they're still told having a hystectomy is their best bet. I beg to differ.

Now, don't get me wrong. If you're suffering from uterine or ovarian cancer, a hysterectomy is mandatory—that represents 10 percent of the hysterectomies performed in the United States each year. You also could be forced to have a hysterectomy because of complications from a pregnancy or excessive bleeding. And you could be like my aunt and feel that a hysterectomy will serve you best. Just don't become one of the unfortunate women who choose to have a hysterectomy out of ignorance and later find that you've lost your reproductive organs unnecessarily.

SO HOW DO I TELL MY EMPLOYER?

For some women, communicating with their employer is almost as nerve-racking as determining how they're going to resolve their fibroid dilemma. After all, how will they ever manage without you?

Get a grip, girlfriend, the job was there before you got there and it will probably be there after you leave. But you've only got one body, so let your health be your priority. The good news about fibroids is that they typically don't require emergency treatment, so you've got time to tie up any loose ends before you go out on medical leave and you can schedule your surgery (if that's the option you select) during a slow time of the year, assuming that there is such a thing. Remember, you'll be out for a significant period (four to six weeks) only if you choose to have a myomectomy or hysterectomy. And even if you choose one of those options, you'll be back before you know it saying, "Gosh, the time away was way too short." Believe me, I know!

Before you schedule anything, contact your insurance provider to find out which services are covered and to confirm the procedures. Some insurance providers require that you contact them ahead of time to approve your surgery and hospital stay. Ask the company directly and then double-check the information with your physician. These details are important because any mistake on your part could result in your receiving a hefty hospital bill, and that's the last thing you want. So make it easy on yourself and get the facts on your health coverage.

Once you find out about your coverage and have scheduled a date, let your employer in on the good news: ASAP. (Yes, good news: you're taking action so you can get the relief you deserve, and that's good.) Start by talking to your manager, who will probably tell you to have a conversation with the company's human resource department. If you don't feel comfortable telling your boss all of the gory details, simply say that you need to have surgery and it will require that you be out of the office for four to six weeks (for a myomectomy or hysterectomy). Then

Conventional Remedies At-a-Glance

Treatment	Description	Time for Procedure	Pros/Cons	Price Ranges	Success Rates	Recovery Time
Wait and See	Follow up with your physician every six months to track the size of the fibroids.	Your gynecologist will review the status of your fibroids every six months.	Enables you to avoid acting prematurely. Least expensive approach.	$5 to $15 copayment for checkup	Varies—some women don't even know they have them.	N/A
Drugs	Birth control pills, GnRH-based drugs (Lupron and Synarel) are used to treat cramps and heavy bleeding. GnRH-based drugs are given before surgery to reduce fibroid size. Birth control pills are used to regulate menstrual cycle, alleviate cramps, and	GnRHs are usually prescribed for three months.	Noninvasive, non-surgical technique. Drugs have different side effects. GnRH drugs cause menopause-like symptoms.	If not covered by insurance, GnRH drugs can cost $300 a treatment.	Varies. Lupron or Synarel have been known for temporary shrinkage of up to 50% over a three-month period.	N/A

Treatment	Description	Time for Procedure	Pros/Cons	Price Ranges	Success Rates	Recovery Time
	control heavy bleeding.					
Myolysis (Myoma Coagulation)	High-frequency electric currents and laser energy is used to destroy the fibroid.	Thirty minutes	Short hospital stay and recovery time. Destroyed fibroids do not regrow. Possible complications from surgery. Could affect fertility. New fibroids can develop.	Actual procedure costs compare to a hysterectomy or myomectomy but because of shorter hospital stay may come out cheaper in long run.	Goldfarb (doctor who introduced procedure to U.S.) claims 80 percent of his patients had no subsequent symptoms but research on this procedure is limited.	Outpatient hospital procedure. Can return to work within one to two weeks.
Uterine Artery Embolization	Tiny particles (polyvinyl alcohol) are inserted through the groin into the uterine artery to block the blood flow and eventually shrink the fibroids.	One hour	Short recovery. Although immediate improvements can occur, maximum recovery seen in four to six months. Not recommended for women who want to have children.	$6,000–9,000	7 out of 10 UAE patients report positive results.	One week

Treatment	Description	Time for Procedure	Pros/Cons	Price Ranges	Success Rates	Recovery Time
Myomec-tomy	The surgical removal of the fibroid(s) while leaving the uterus intact.	Two to three hours depending on the number of fibroids.	Fertility is preserved. External and internal scars may occur. Fibroids may return.	Approximately $800 less than a hysterectomy.		Requires a three- to four-day hospital stay and four to six weeks home stay for recovery.
Hystererc-tomy	Surgical procedure that removes the uterus.	Two hours	Fibroids will never recur because there is no uterus. Women suffer the same side effects as if they entered menopause (if ovaries are removed as well) and there could be mental and physical side effects that result from not having a uterus.	$1,000–3,000	100%. Uterine fibroids never recur.	Requires a three- to four-day hospital stay and four to six weeks home stay for recovery.

assure your boss that you will do everything you can to help things run smoothly in your absence and request suggestions that will enable you to make that happen. Any boss that has your best interest at heart will express sympathy for your situation and offer support. A poor manager will only be concerned about the workload, which will get done whether you're around or not—I promise. If the scenario results in the latter response, don't take it personally. Your primary concern is YOU, and the only thing you need to ensure is that you've conducted yourself in a respectful, professional manner demonstrating your desire to promote a smooth transition during your absence and upon your return.

The firm's human resource department can clarify any additional concerns you have about your health insurance, explain the company policy regarding medical leave, and tell you about disability coverage if it applies. Basically, short-term disability is paid by your employer to the state and it allows you to receive 66⅔ percent of your salary for a maximum of six weeks. You may be eligible for short-term disability if your treatment requires an extended recovery period. But you'll need a note from your physician indicating that you require surgery as well as the length of time you're expected to need for recovery. It's not required that you reveal why you're having surgery, but if you want disability then the doctor is required to write in the type of surgery that you're having on a questionnaire and that form is then submitted to your employer. In addition, you will need a release from your doctor, stating that you are well enough for work, when you return to the office. So don't forget to ask for this form from your physician and keep a copy for yourself for your records.

Employer To-Do List

✔ Decide on treatment method for your fibroids.

Date:_____ Time: _____

✔ Confirm with insurance provider that the option you chose is covered.

Date:_____ Time: _____

✔ Schedule treatment date with your physician.

Date:_____ Time: _____

✔ Let your boss know that you need to be out for medical reasons and tell how long you need to be out.

Date:_____ Time: _____

✔ Talk to company human resources department and confirm insurance and disability coverage.

Date:_____ Time: _____

✔ Get a note from your doctor confirming surgery date and leave time.

Date:_____ Time: _____

✔ Tell a coworker that you need to be out and ask that they keep you informed about company news.

Date:_____ Time: _____

✔ Schedule a follow-up meeting with your boss so you can discuss how your work will be handled in your absence.

Date:_____ Time: _____

✔ Schedule a meeting with the person who will be taking on your responsibilities in your absence.

Date:_____ Time: _____

✔ Call in once every two weeks to let your colleagues know how you're doing and to get an update on them.

Date:_____ Time: _____

✔ Secure a release from your doctor, stating that you are well enough for work, when you're ready to go back to the office.

Date:_____ Time: _____

6 Au Naturel Remedies

Evaluating Nontraditional Fibroid-Fighting Alternatives

Whether or not the medical community likes to acknowledge it, an increasing number of Black women are turning to alternative, or holistic, medicine like nutritional therapy, herbal medicines and even Chinese acupuncture in an effort to find relief from their fibroids. Russell Harrison, a master herbalist for more than 20 years in Pasadena, California, says that since he started practicing holistic medicine in 1978, hundreds of women with uterine fibroids have come to him for treatment.

"Most have gone through traditional methods and are dissatisfied," he says about his clients. And some Sisters say they are getting positive results from their unconventional therapy, even claiming that their fibroids shrank.

—Ebony Magazine, March 1998

First of all, let me remind you that using home-grown medicine (or "alternative" remedies, in today's terms) is nothing new for us. "Black women in America relied on plant medicines for healing long before it was fashionable, but many of us are just discovering this natural healing art," writes Ziba Kashef in her book *Like a Natural Woman: The Black Woman's Guide to Alternative Healing* (Kensington, $23.). That's right, we've been brewing up natural healing stews from leaves, stems, barks, roots, and flowers since the beginning of time, either because we have been denied access to traditional medical offerings or because we truly believe that natural remedies are best. You remember how your grandmother would use the aloe vera plant to treat burns, and force you to take castor oil or cod liver for colds. Those concoctions were handed down to us from our ancestors who brought some of the herbs and traditions surrounding their use (such as wild yam to treat female problems such as menstrual cramps) right from the Motherland. West Africans used plants as seasoning for foods, healing agents, magical preparations, and even as poisons. With some guidance from Native Americans as well as their own insights, when the Africans arrived in the United States they were able to continue their healing traditions by associating specific plants with the curing of certain diseases on the basis of the plants' fragrance and appearance.

Some of these notions served as "remarkable natural healing tools," adds Kashef. "Used properly, herbs can affect mild and serious illness without troublesome side effects." Results from herbal treatments have, to some degree, been verified. Certain herbs held up under close scrutiny when tested in clinical trials conducted by researchers at the Centre for Scientific Research in Ghana.[1] In addition to Africans and African Americans, Indians, Native Americans, and the Chinese use herbal medicine as a regular component of the healing process. Further, approximately 80 percent of the entire world population relies on herbal remedies for prevention or cure, and one-quarter of Western conventional pharmaceutical medicine is derived from some of the same herbs and minerals used in developing natural remedies.[2]

There is, however, a big difference between herbal remedies and Western medicine. The combinations used in pharmaceutical drugs have gone through controlled lab testing and peer review studies and have been approved by the United States Food and Drug Administration (FDA). Alternative remedies are unregulated and have not gone through similar testing procedures. As a result, you can't be sure that over-the-counter remedies have the right amount of active ingredients to be effective. These products may be contaminated with other herbs, may contain ingredients that aren't listed on the label, and are often very expensive. In addition, since there is no government regulation of the distribution of natural drugs or natural practitioners, the industry is full of quacks (practitioners who knowingly offer phony cures). Even the most highly regarded natural practitioners can't seem to consistently predict outcomes when natural remedies are used. They offer no guarantees, arguing that each patient's health issues are unique and treatments must be customized for that individual's set of circumstances.

Many medical doctors are uncomfortable with the unpredictability factor that is inherent in using natural remedies and do not support their use. "I don't recommend natural remedies because there is no clinical data to support the efficacy of over the counter compounds. If you want to be a human guinea pig, go to a health store and buy anything that they recommend. None of these herbal compounds has ever undergone scientific investigation to develop a dose-response curve. One doesn't know how much to take and what effects will occur. It's basically experimental," insists Yvonne S. Thornton, M.D., M.P.H. "When these naturalists can give me a dose-response curve and a history of the drugs they're selling as well as how these substances react with other drugs then I'll hear them out. When patients go to health food stores they are taking their health in their own hands. There is a Food and Drug Administration out there that's for everyone's best interest. . . . For every one or ten testimonials from patients [in support of natural remedies], there are thirty or forty patients that have not obtained the same results and some have even gotten negative results. That's why it's important to have nonbiased studies." Dr. Obiakor agrees: "Until good scientific controlled studies have been done with these elements to prove their efficacy, I do not recommend them. I'm not saying they're not effective but there haven't been any scientific large scale studies to prove whether they work or are harmful."

As far as the treatment of fibroids is concerned, "the jury is still out on this one," admits Sir Abdulla Smithford, a naturopathic physician. "There aren't any clinical data to support that natural remedies affect the growth of fibroids," he says. Other naturopathic physicians also concede that uterine fibroids have consistently eluded successful treatment. "Women who are seeking an alternative to the drug or surgical treatment of uterine fibroids will not find an easy, reliable alternative to shrink the tumors within natural medicine," according to the *Women's Encyclopedia of Natural Medicine: Alternative Therapies and Integrative Medicine* (Keats, 1999, $24.95) by Tori Hudson, N.D. At best, fibroid sufferers can expect some relief from symptoms such as excessive bleeding, pressure, pelvic pain, and backaches. They may also experience some slowed growth of their fibroids that could prevent additional problems. However, there have been only minimal results when natural remedies are used for the treatment of larger fibroids. And even though there have been some exceptions, "the results are very inconsistent and random," admits Hudson, who says that more likely than not, symptomatic large fibroids will probably require some kind of interventional treatment.

So does this mean we should totally disregard the use of natural remedies for the treatment of fibroids? The short answer is: it depends. If your fibroids are small or if you want to explore another possibility before opting for a hysterectomy, you may decide to try a natural approach. Just be sure to get educated about herbs before you start taking them, including knowing how much to take and for how long you should take them, because some over-the-counter remedies can actually be toxic or can worsen the symptoms that you're trying to cure. Herbs such as black cohosh or goldenseal, for example, can be toxic if taken in large amounts. Others, such as kava kava or horsetail, can be harmful if taken for long periods of time. Avoid taking any herbal formulas until you consult a licensed herbalist and your physician. Dr. Deidre S. Maccannon of Michigan works with her patients who want to explore natural remedies: "I encourage my patients to talk to me about alternative medicine. That way I can research it and monitor them." Even with your physician's support, you should use your own judgment. If after evaluating the results over a few days or weeks, your medical doctor can offer no proof that the treatment is effective and you think the treatment is unsuccessful, or if you start getting unexpected or unwanted side effects, stop using it immediately.

This chapter will highlight some of the more common natural remedies for fibroids by detailing their use, side effects, inconsistencies, and interactions with other medications. In addition, this section will also show you how to tell a qualified practitioner from a quack. Use the information here to familiarize yourself with the industry's offerings and help you determine whether natural remedies are for you. I also encourage you to do additional research on any option you plan to explore, because new information is always being released and you can never be too careful when it comes to your health.

WHAT'S A NATURAL REMEDY?

The term *natural* has been misused in questionable advertising claims, according to Michael Castleman, author of *Nature's Cures: From Acupressure & Aromatherapy to Walking & Yoga, the Ultimate Guide to the Best Scientifically Proven, Drug-Free Healing Methods* (Bantam, $6.99). Traditionally, *natural* means substances that have not been tampered with scientifically. In conventional medicine, scientists isolate the active ingredient of an herb or plant and leave out all of the other substances that they feel don't contribute to healing. But natural remedies use the whole product whether it's a plant or an herb. The term *natural*, at times, has also included healthy habits such as exercising and diet management as strategies to treat disease.

For our purposes, *natural* refers to treatments that are outside of conventional medicine. But even that can still be confusing because the distinction between natural and conventional is becoming blurred even by members of the medical field. There are a number of "conventional" physicians that include a large range of alternative therapies—including homeopathy, acupuncture, and herbal remedies—in their treatment plan. They're also prescribing alternative therapies such as a healthy diet, meditation, massage, yoga, and dietary supplements to their patients. In addition, as Castleman points out, there are certain treatments such as biofeedback, vision therapy, lucid dreaming, and bright light therapy that appear to be alternative remedies but are actually treatment options that were derived from conventional medicine. Finally, the school of thought that considers herbal remedies as "alternative" and conventional medicine as "mainstream" doesn't really hold up, because the majority of people around the world have relied on natural remedies since the beginning of time. Conventional medicine is actually less widely used and much newer than natural remedies. "If healing arts were judged by worldwide numerical support or duration of use, many 'alternative' therapies would be 'mainstream,' and vice versa," insists Castleman.

So how should you consider these treatments in relation to your own fibroid condition? Experts suggest that you look at these natural remedies as a complement to your "conventional" treatment plan, not a replacement. Natural therapies such as diet management, exercise, touch, positive thinking, and other healing arts fill in certain gaps where conventional medicine is concerned. Use natural cures "to enhance your well-being and prevent illness," advises Castleman.

Also, don't rely on any natural remedy as a guaranteed cure or as a substitute for getting a diagnosis from a traditional physician. Some people practice natural treatment plans without getting a bill of good health from a medical doctor, and that's not recommended. Getting a prompt diagnosis and regular checkups is key for the management of any health condition regardless of the treatment option you select. "If you have a particular problem go see your doctor or health care professional first," advises Sir Abdulla Smithford. Then if you decide to try a natural remedy, "work with a medical professional that understands your need to work from a natural point of view and ask him to help you get that type of treatment," he suggests.

Queen Afua, a nationally renowned herbalist, holistic health specialist, and author of *Heal Thyself for Health and Longevity* (A&B, $9.95) and *SACRED WOMAN: A guide to healing the feminine body, mind and spirit* (Ballantine, $28), agrees. "Now the doctors are studying and are going in the direction [of natural healing] so that they stay connected to those [patients] who are striving to be more independent. I have doctors that have come to see me for wellness. I also have doctors that I recommend for people to go out and have their full examination," she says. "If someone is seeing a doctor they should continue seeing their doctor and if that patient takes on a natural lifestyle then both of them will see an improvement every month," Afua insists.

Finally, remember that "herbs are medicine. Natural doesn't mean safe, it just means that the remedy can be safer than a pharmaceutical option," states Smithford. "People feel [natural remedies are] probably safer because they believe they have less side effects [than conventional medicine]. But everything that is natural can, beyond a certain dosage, act as a medicinal agent in the human system. In other words, if you eat an excess of onions they can also induce toxicity. Natural remedies can still cause side effects which can result in medical conditions." Again, medical supervision is essential when using natural products.

NATURAL FIBROID FIXES?

If you think you can stir up some plants and leaves in your blender for a fast fibroid remedy, think again. There is no one natural fix for fibroids and the results, if any, certainly won't come fast. The regimen that most practitioners prescribe as treatment for fibroids is strict: the elimination of all flesh foods (such as red meat, chicken, or fish), junk food, dairy products, and alcohol; participation in regular meditation and exercise programs; and the intake of organic foods and certain herbs and teas. The products for such a regimen can be costly, and the process requires strict discipline. Further, the results could take months, maybe even years, and may not appear at all. But, according to proponents of natural remedies, when holistic treatments are successful, they're a permanent fix, because they totally repair the body and whatever condition that caused the fibroids to grow is eliminated or repaired.

Just what herbal remedies do experts suggest for the treatment of fibroids? The list is a long one. Again, these remedies are more for managing the symptoms associated with fibroids rather than the myomas themselves. Hudson says that her objective in treating women with large fibroids is to alleviate some of the symptoms, try to find ways to make the patient more comfortable until menopause (when the fibroids will probably shrink), and identify situations where conventional treatment is the most appropriate remedy. "One aspect of being a naturopathic physician is to more fully educate patients about their health and their health problems so they can make informed decisions about their health care," she adds.

Use the chart on the following pages, which highlights the more popular remedies for fibroid symptoms, to increase your knowledge about herbal treatments. Be aware that this listing is in no way complete and is not an endorsement of any of the herbs that are included. Remember, you really do use natural remedies at your own risk. Also note that some of these treatments, even though they may be popularly publicized, have harsh side effects or could be dangerous if taken along with other herbs or medications. Regardless of what your herbalist recommends, research the drug's effectiveness and side effects with an independent source. In addition, track your symptoms and discontinue using any remedy that makes you feel worse.

HOW DO YOU USE THESE REMEDIES?

Herbal remedies can be used in a variety of ways, both internally and externally. According to Kashef, the most effective method for you depends on your body chemistry, the herb, and the condition you want to treat. Here's how she explains the various uses:

Internal

Capsule: This is the best form for potent herbs that require small dosages or will be taken for long periods of time. Under these conditions, capsules are convenient and help you avoid contact with bitter-tasting herbs. You can purchase capsules at a pharmacy or health food

Herbs said to . . .	Shrink	Detoxify	Alleviate Cramps	Manage Bleeding	Menstrual Problems	Warning
Astragalus					X (also for vaginal infections)	None known
Aurum muriaticum	X					Should only take if there is no heavy bleeding or particular discomfort
Berth Root				X		
Black Cohosh					X	Can worsen cramps and make uterine cells divide. Avoid during pregnancy.
Black Haw			X			Sedative
Blue Cohosh					X	Can increase blood pressure and resrtict blood vessels leading to the heart. Unsafe during pregnancy.
Blue Flag		X				
Chamomile	X					May cause an allergic reaction.

Herbs said to . . .	Shrink	Detoxify	Alleviate Cramps	Manage Bleeding	Menstrual Problems	Warning
Chaste tree berry, or Vitex agnuscastus	X			X		Causes uterine cells to divide. May make birth control pills ineffective. May cause skin irritation or stomach-aches.
Chuan xiong				X		Regulates bleeding according to the amount taken. Too much can cause uterine bleeding. Should take under the guidance of a Chinese herbal practitioner.
Cinnamon				X		
Cramp Bark			X	X		
Dandelion		X				Diuretic effect. Shouldn't be used if 'cold' symptoms are present.
Dong quai			X			Should avoid this if you have heavy menstrual bleeding.

Herbs said to . . .	Shrink	Detoxify	Alleviate Cramps	Manage Bleeding	Menstrual Problems	Warning
Echinacea	X					Do not use if you have an autoimmune deficiency disorder such as multiple sclerosis or lupus.
Er jow				X		Should take under the guidance of a Chinese herbal practitioner.
Evening Primrose					X	None known
False Unicorn Root				X		
Garlic	X		X			To prevent clotting problems, don't use with anticoagulants (blood thinners) such as Coumadin or aspirin. Can cause stomach upset.
Ginger			X			Consult physician if pregnant or have gallstones. High dose can lower blood pressure.

Herbs said to . . .	Shrink	Detoxify	Alleviate Cramps	Manage Bleeding	Menstrual Problems	Warning
Han lian cao			X			Should take under the guidance of a Chinese herbal practitioner.
Hops			X			Chronic exposure can produce nausea, vomiting, sweating, fever, and skin reactions.
Hydrastinum muriaticum	X					
Lady's Mantle				X		
Licorice			X		X	Can raise blood pressure, particularly if you're on the pill. Only use for four to six weeks.
Motherwort				X		Can make bleeding worse.
Nettle				X		
Partridgeberry			X	X		
Passionflower					X	
Poo Wha				X		Should take under the guidance of a Chinese herbal practitioner.

Herbs said to . . .	Shrink	Detoxify	Alleviate Cramps	Manage Bleeding	Menstrual Problems	Warning
Raspberry Leaves			X			
Sequoia Buds	X					
Shepherd's Purse				X		
Skullcap		X	X			
St. John's Wort			X			Do not combine with other antidepressants. Prolonged use can cause health problems.
White Ash	X					
Wild Yam				X	X	Could cause stomach irritation.
Yarrow	X		X	X		Occasional toxicity.

Sources: Johanna Skilling, *Fibroids: The Complete Guide to Taking Charge of Your Physical, Emotional, and Sexual Well-Being*, 122.
Ziba Kashef, *Like a Natural Woman: The Black Woman's Guide to Alternative Healing*, 80–84.
Dr. Gary Null, *Women's Encyclopedia of Natural Healing*, 95

store. Be sure to look at the expiration date, and keep in mind that because these formulas are unregulated, you can't be completely sure that you're getting the recommended ingredients, but you can consult the salesperson for guidance. You can also make them up yourself by purchasing empty capsules along with the powdered herbs or dried herbal extracts that you can process using a blender or coffee grinder. Powdered herbs are easier to prepare but don't last long. To preserve their potency, store capsules away from heat and light.

Tea: Your own medicinal tea preparation will probably be more effective than over-the-counter teas because those usually lack enough active ingredients to be of any benefit. There are two types of teas. An *infusion* is made by filling a container with a pint of recently boiled water over two tablespoons of dried leaves or flowers with a cover for up to twenty minutes. The leaves are strained out before drinking. Use more herbs if they are fresh. A *decoction* is made by crushing a tougher plant part (roots, barks, stems, and leaves) with a coffee grinder or by hand. Next boil two ounces of the herbs in a pint of water. Then let simmer for twenty minutes up to an hour (depending on the herb) where half of the water should evaporate at this point. Strain out herbs prior to drinking.

When brewing your own teas:

- Use spring or distilled water.
- Use one ounce of herb for every pint of water.
- Confirm the dosage, which could vary from a few tablespoons to a few cups depending on the condition, with a licensed herbalist or physician.
- Try to prepare enough to store for at least three days.

Tea for Uterine Fibroids

1 teaspoon of burdock root	½ teaspoon mullein leaves
1 teaspoon of cramp bark	½ teaspoon cleavers leaves
1 teaspoon of motherwort leaves	½ teaspoon ginger rhizome
1 teaspoon wild yam rhizome	1 quart water
½ teaspoon prickly ash bark	

Combine all ingredients in a pot and bring to boil. Then lower flame and let mixture simmer for a few minutes. Next turn heat off and let sit for 20 minutes. Strain brew into a container. Drink a minimum of two cups per day. You can also take in pill form or as a tincture. You may have to drink this brew for several months for full benefit.

Source: Kathi Keville, *Herbs for Health and Healing: A Drug-Free Guide to Prevention and Cure* (Rodale, $27.95).

Tincture: A concentrated version of essential ingredients is extracted when cut or powdered herbs are combined with alcohol (e.g., grain alcohol) or glycerin and then preserved for a four-week period. You can purchase tinctures in stores or make them yourself by combining one part of chopped or ground herb with two parts alcohol or other solvent in a tightly covered jar. Over the storing period, shake the jar daily and then strain it. The liquid should then be funneled into small labeled bottles for storage. If the herbs you're using are bitter-tasting or potent, or if you plan on using them for a long period of time, tinctures are a great alternative.

Extract: These substances are much more concentrated and more potent than tinctures. When using extracts, the dosages aren't more than a few drops.

External

Oil: Typically derived from sweet-smelling herbs such as lavender and rose, oils are highly concentrated preparations that can be used in bath water for added relaxation or in a diffuser to disperse the aroma throughout your environment. You can also use oils as a lubricant for massages. Just be careful, because large doses of essential oils can irritate the skin and may even be toxic. Be sure to properly dilute them before using them.

To mix up your own essential oils:

- Grind 2 cups of fresh or dried herbs.
- Mix with 4 cups of oil (try sesame or olive oil).
- Let it sit for an hour or boil for an hour.
- Strain through a strainer that has a coffee filter in it.
- Put strained contents in a bottle for storing.

Compress: Soak a cloth in diluted tincture, diluted oil, or herbal tea. Wring it out and then lay the cloth on the problem area. This process is particularly effective for cramps, joint or muscle pain, or headaches.

Castor Oil Packs

Castor oil should be heated on the stove to a warm but bearable temperature. Then saturate a cloth with the castor oil and place it over the abdomen (breasts if you have fibroids in those areas) while you're lying flat on your back. Next cover the cloth with plastic wrap and place a larger towel on top. Then place a hot water bottle or heating pad on top of the towel and cover with a large towel. Relax for forty-five minutes to two hours. Once the treatment is removed, massage the area by manipulating your fingers in a circular motion. You should repeat this process daily for ten days and take a break for two days. The procedure should not be done while you're on your period, so if you start menstruating stop the treatment and resume when your cycle ends. After you've used the castor oil packs for three cycles, break for a month, and then resume the treatment if symptoms persist.

Liniment: This preparation is rubbed directly on the skin. Place finely chopped dried or fresh herbs in a jar and cover with rubbing alcohol. Allow to settle for at least two weeks while shaking the jar every two days. Next strain the substance through a coffee filter into another jar and add a label. Good for inflammations such as arthritis.

Poultice: To use herbs in this form, moisten the powdered herb with tincture, herbal tea, or hot water. Insert the mixture into the fold of a piece of gauze and then place on the problem area. Used to soothe bruises and draw out toxins through the skin.

Salve: Make this thick healing preparation by adding one part beeswax to four parts of warmed infused oil that is stored in a covered jar. Another alternative is to add powdered herbs to hot lard. Of course, allow the substance to cool before applying it to skin. Salves are used to treat topical skin irritations.

CHOOSING A NATURAL PRACTITIONER

If you're considering going the natural route for your treatment, you'll first need to distinguish a qualified practitioner from a quack. Here are some suggestions for picking a practitioner that's right for you:

Do your research. Review magazines, newspapers, and other sources that contain information about natural health care. Also search the Internet for natural health–related sites. In addition, sign up for any free newsletters or webzines that can provide you with insight. The key here is to properly evaluate the sources as well as the accuracy and reliability of the information that you're reading before you base your decision on that source.

Contact governing organizations. Depending on the type of service and the state, there may be a governing body. If so, you can check if a particular practitioner is a member of that organization and is following proper guidelines. They can probably tell you whether the practitioner is practicing legally, has the right credentials, and has had any complaints filed against him (refer to your local Better Business Bureau as well).

Check membership in professional organizations. Membership in professional organizations is optional and is not required for anyone to legally practice. However, a practitioner's lack of membership may indicate a lower level of interest in the profession. Some professional associations can provide insight on a practitioner's reputation, training, experience, specialization, and education. However, be aware that many professional groups do not confirm a member's credentials.

Contact reputable schools on nontraditional therapies. These institutions have a selection of professionals among their faculty as well as a long list of graduates that they refer. Using a practitioner that teaches at an institution may indicate a high level of interest as well as an awareness of the latest developments in the field.

Get referrals from people you trust. Turn to your family doctor or a trusted health practitioner for a reliable referral. Generally, health professionals have a long list of contacts in various aspects of the medical field so they can help you make a connection. Also ask your family, friends, and coworkers to pass on contact information for any natural practitioners that they liked. Even if you don't go with the ones that you were offered, you'll still have a sense of what qualities you find important so you can choose a practitioner on your own.

Another Natural Remedies Regimen for Fibroids

Change diet to reduce your intake of estrogen-generating foods such as meat, eggs, cheese, and other dairy products. Also, limit coffee, sugar, and alcohol intake.

Eat dark leafy green vegetables; whole grains; protein-enriched foods such as tempeh fish, tofu, organically raised chicken; herbal teas and fresh fruits. Drink Spirulina Green Tea daily.

Spirulina Green Tea

Combine the following ingredients:

1 pound spirulina	6 ounces powdered apple pectin
½ pound bee pollen	6 ounces granulated lecithin

Combine (using a blender) 1 to 2 tablespoons of the mixture in a cup of fruit juice such as pineapple or orange juice. Store the balance of mix in the freezer until ready to use.

Take two Chaparral capsules three times a day for three months.

Chaparral Capsules

Insert in a capsule:

1 part pau d'arco powder	1 part yellow dock root powder
1 chaparral powder	1 part vitex (chaste berry) powder

Drink three to four cups of Liver Tea Cleanser or Immune Cleanser Tea every day.

Liver Tea Cleanser

1 part yellow dock root	1 part Oregon grape root
2 parts wild yam root	2 parts burdock root
1 part dandelion root	1 part vitex (chaste berry)

Add cinnamon, ginger, sassafras and orange peel to taste. To use, add 4 to 6 tablespoons of mix per quart of cold water. Then put contents in a covered pot and bring to a simmer over low heat for 20 minutes. Remove from heat and allow to infuse for another 20 minutes. Strain and drink.

Immune Cleanser

1 part yellow dock root	1 part astragalus
1 part ginger	1 part licorice root
3 parts dandelion root	1 part vitex (chaste berry)
1 part dong quai	4 parts pau d'arco
2 parts burdock root	

Add cinnamon, ginger, sassafras, orange peel, and stevia to taste.
Use 4 to 6 tablespoons of herb mixture per quart of cold water. Then allow to simmer in a covered pot over low heat for 20 minutes.

Remove from heat and allow to infuse for another 20 minutes. Strain and drink.

Take sitz baths five nights a week.

Sitz Bath—Helps reduce blood stagnation and blocked energy in the pelvic area by enabling the blood vessels to dilate and constrict.

Two large metal buckets that can comfortably hold your buttocks but can fit in your bathtub.

Fill one with hot water and one with cold.

Add herbal tea such as nettle or raspberry to hot water.

Drop ice cubes in cold water.

Sit in hot water (which should not be hot enough to burn you) for several minutes.

Then transfer yourself into the cold water bucket for several minutes (right before you start to feel comfortable with the temperature).

Then switch back to the hot water bucket.

Repeat this process five to six times for several times during the week.

After baths use castor oil packs (see castor oil packs side bar) and Vaginal Bolus II five nights during the week.

Vaginal Bolus II

1 part yellow dock root	½ part black walnut hull powder
1 part chaparra leaf powder	1 to 2 drops of essential oil of
1 part goldenseal root powder	myrrh and/or tea tree oil
3 parts slippery elm bark powder	1 cup coconut oil
1 part witch hazel bark powder	

Run ingredients through a grinder.

Melt coconut oil in a saucepan over low heat. When oil is completely melted, remove from heat and stir in powdered ingredients. Mix until you get a thick paste that you're able to roll into "Tootsie Roll" shapes that are the width of your small finger. Insert bolus as far up into your vagina as possible.

Source: Rosemary Gladstar, *Herbal Healing for Women: Simple Remedies for Women of All Ages* (Fireside, 1993), 162.

ARE NATURAL REMEDIES RIGHT FOR YOU?

Only you can answer that question. Remember, if your fibroids are large; are causing medical problems that may require fast treatment such as extreme pain, excessive bleeding, or infertility; or have been found to be cancerous (which occurs in less than 1 percent of women), conventional remedies offer better options because natural treatments are more for long-term treatment. Alternatively, if time is on your side and you're ready to exercise the discipline that natural regimens require, then perhaps you could try herbs and other alternatives alone or use them along with other treatments. Just know their limitations, and have a budget in mind, because these treatments won't be covered by your employer-sponsored insurance plan—so you'll be footing the bill. Also be aware that even though there are numerous sources touting the success stories of fibroid sufferers who have been miraculously cured by nontraditional therapies, the majority of those claims are unfounded. And no matter what treatment you decide to use, don't make any moves unless you bring your consumer smarts along for the ride. Talk to others about their experiences with a particular treatment or practitioner, ask lots of questions, and if something sounds too good to be true, it's probably a scam.

Conventional versus Natural Approaches to Treatment

If you're wondering how conventional and natural medicine differ, this chart illustrates the benefits and shortcomings of each approach. But again, don't view either method as your only alternative; the two views can complement each other and provide you with a more complete treatment plan.

Conventional Medicine	Natural Medicine
Base theory: Eliminate the problem.	Base theory: Aid body in healing itself.
Emphasizes diagnosis.	Emphasizes disease prevention.
Views your fibroids as a specific problem.	Views the mind and body as one, the bodymind, and looks at your fibroids as the symptom of some underlying larger issue.
Uses a "one size fits all" approach to treat fibroid issues.	Customized treatment approaches are designed for each individual.
Body is looked at as essentially a machine that develops diseases as a result of broken or poorly operating parts.	Body is looked at as a living microcosm of the universe that develops disease when its forces become unbalanced.
Efforts tackle diseases.	Efforts restore harmony between the mind and body.
Patient is a passive participant in receipt of a "quick fix."	Patient is an active participant in activities that promote self-repair and self-healing.
Office typically sterile and cold.	Treatment atmosphere typically calm and relaxing.
Primary remedies include medication, surgery, and radiation.	Primary remedies include dietary changes, exercise, stress management, herbal medicines, and social support.
Remedies can have side effects during or after procedures.	Remedies typically do not have side effects during or after procedure.
Remedies are temporary unless an invasive procedure is used.	Works best for symptoms such as cramping or bleeding.
Can treat all sizes of fibroids.	Better for treating smaller fibroids.
Remedies work relatively quickly.	Remedies take a long time (months or years) to work.
Follow-up is limited after surgical treatment.	Requires ongoing interaction with practitioner.

Conventional Medicine	Natural Medicine
Lifestyle change not required.	Lifestyle change required.
Has a track record to prove results and is based on peer-reviewed studies.	No track record, comparative studies, or trials for treating fibroids.
Drugs and procedures are regulated by the U.S. Food and Drug Administration.	Not regulated by the government.
Treatments are covered by insurance.	Treatments are not covered by insurance.
Concentration on disease.	Concentration on the human experience of disease, illnesses.
Concentration on pain.	Concentration on the human experience of pain, suffering.
Cure is the objective.	Healing and the development of the individual's experience of physical, mental, and spiritual wholeness is the objective.

Sources: Michael Castleman, *Nature's Cures: From Acupressure & Aromatherapy to Walking & Yoga, the Ultimate Guide to the Best Scientifically Proven, Drug-Free Healing Methods* (Bantam, 1996, $6.99) xxv, and Johanna Skilling, *Fibroids: The Complete Guide to Taking Charge of Your Physical, Emotional, and Sexual Well-Being* (New York: Marlowe & Company, 2000), 119.

7

The F-Word

Managing Your Fibroids Through Your Food Intake

I saw a special on television and had been hearing a lot about natural ways of living and how foods affect the body and cause fibroids, tumors, and so on and so forth. I believed what I heard; however, I kept eating meats and drinking the dairy even though I am highly allergic to it. I was so conditioned that I tried to convince myself that the food I was eating wasn't affecting my fibroids. Still, they continued to grow.

After a while I just had to stop eating those things. When I wasn't eating meat the fibroids would subside, but once I went back to my poor diet they came back. I started reading more and more on alternative foods and the different ways of taking care of my body, but it was a real struggle for me for years. I really had to fight to let go of [the bad foods] because it was like any addiction. Finally, sometime last year, I completely changed my diet. Now I'm less agitated and the fibroids are gone.

—Queen Bast Nebt-Het, Age 41

Girlfriend, you've heard the saying that you are what you eat. Well, that's especially true when it comes to fibroids. In fact, you'll never experience the full benefit of any treatment you choose unless you make some necessary changes in your food intake. "So many African American women have fibroids because we have the lowest capacity to tolerate the 'Standard American Diet' and, due to occupying the lowest stratum on the social totem pole, are also the most stressed out," states Rosa Kincaid, M.D., a family practitioner and student of Chinese medicine, African and Western herbology, and nutrition for more than thirty years. She says the key to being fibroid-free is to reduce stress (we'll address this later) and eliminate our "toxic diet."

Other experts agree. According to Queen Afua, "[Fibroids] are developed and caused by impure blood, unbalanced diet, and constipation. They grow from a heavy fat diet of flesh, such as pork, beef, and chicken (animals that are shot up with hormones) as well as the by-products of flesh such as eggs, cheese, and milk. The tumors are further cultivated from an emotional and stressful life." Queen Afua says that we really are what we eat and has observed over her thirty years of practice that women whose diets are high in flesh and junk food have heavier menstruation and are more likely to have fibroids. "Toxic foods create an environment for wombs to grow tumors," she contends. "I also found that if a woman has a tumor removed and she doesn't change her diet the tumors usually return within one to two years following surgery. Healthy habits can prevent surgery."

In *The Woman's Encyclopedia of Natural Healing: The New Healing Techniques of 100 Leading Alternative Health Practitioners* by Dr. Gary Null, nutritionist Gracia Perlstein also advocates dietary changes as a primary strategy for tackling fibroids. "Research shows that an over-fatty diet increases estrogen in the diet," Perlstein says. By now we know that excess estrogen makes fibroids grow. Women that are leaner have a less potent variation of estrogen. Conversely, women with more fat tissues store more estrogen at more potent levels. In addition, girls and women that are overweight have higher levels of free-flowing estrogen since their body's capacity to bind estrogen with substances in the blood is diminished. This free-flowing estrogen in certain women feeds fibroids.

It's no wonder we sisters make the perfect camping grounds for these menacing myomas. "Overweight women produce more estrogen,"[1] Perlstein explains. So not only does a bad diet promote weight gain, but some experts believe fat cells also affect fibroid growth. The theory states that a woman's body fat converts the male hormone androgen (which is present in small amounts in all females) into more estrogen[2]—the very hormone that makes fibroids grow. Since black women carry more weight than their white counterparts, they're also more likely to produce estrogen in excess and that may partially explain their higher propensity to have fibroids as well.

According to the Third National Health and Nutrition Examination Survey, half of all African American women are obese, exceeding their ideal weight by 10 to 20 percent. That's bad news because an Oxford study found that the risk of developing fibroids appears to increase steadily as a woman's weight increases.[3] "The overall risk of fibroids rose roughly 21% for each 20-pound increase in weight. . . . Women weighing 154 pounds or more had almost a threefold increased risk compared with women weighing less than 110 pounds," writes Nelson H. Stringer, author of *Uterine Fibroids: What Every Woman Needs to Know*.

As proof, Stringer points out that the average weight of his laparoscopic myomectomy patients is 155 pounds, and he insists that "the most important lifestyle change you can make is to start a low-fat diet and reduce your weight. Starting a regular exercise program will help you decrease your body fat. These lifestyle alterations will not make a fibroid vanish, but they may slow further growth of the fibroid and produce other important health benefits as well."

If you want to attempt to decrease the size of your fibroids or at least prevent them from getting any larger, try eliminating red meat, dairy products, poultry, hydrogenated and saturated fats, alcohol and other recreational drugs, fried foods, coffee, and refined or processed foods.[4] Although many highly refined, nutrient-poor foods such as cookies, french fries, potato chips, white bread, candy, and pasta are common in the American diet, "this diet puts a woman at risk for fibroid tumors as well as endometriosis and breast cancer," writes Christiane Northrup, M.D., author of *Women's Bodies, Women's Wisdom: Creating Physical and Emotional Health and Healing* (Bantam, $18.95).

But knowing what things to eliminate won't help unless you have a long list of healthy substitutes. This chapter will provide you with a wide selection of fibroid-fighting foods along with some tasty recipes, so you can plan for upcoming dishes, and suggested vitamin supplements. In addition, the chapter concludes with a food diary so you can keep better track of the meals you eat on a daily basis.

FIBROID-FIGHTING FOODS

According to Northrup, "A woman who changes from a highly refined, nutrient-poor diet to a diet rich in fruits, vegetables, and other foods will often experience decreased bleeding, lessened bloating, and even a decrease in the size of her fibroids." She recommends women assess whether they are experiencing any significant results after a three-month trial period. During this time, dairy foods, animal products, processed foods, refined sugar, and flour products should be completely eliminated and replaced with meals containing plenty of leafy green vegetables, soy products, whole foods, fresh fruits, and natural organic products. After the trial period, you will have at least succeeded in improving your eating habits. "Many women are eager to try this approach first, knowing that they can have surgery later if the regimen does not work out," adds Northrup.

Since some theories suggest that fibroids are caused by poor liver function, Dr. Pookrum recommends eating bitter vegetables such as turnip and mustard greens, endive, and escarole to nourish this organ. These foods will also aid in the functioning of the gallbladder. You should also eat fish (mackerel or salmon), nuts, and seeds (flaxseeds) to boost essential fatty acids.

Need other suggestions? Try these:

WHOLE GRAINS

"I strongly recommend the use of certain whole grains such as millet, buckwheat, oats and rice," writes Dr. Susan Lark, M.D., author of *Fibroid Tumors & Endometriosis Self Help Book* (Celestial Arts, $16.95). Whole grains contain vitamin B and vitamin E. These agents positively affect the ovaries and liver to promote a healthy hormonal balance and reduce excessive estrogen levels. The fiber content of whole grains also helps regulate bowel movements so that excessive estrogen, dietary fat, cholesterol, and other toxins are swiftly eliminated—good news for the one in two fibroid sufferers that have constipation complaints.[5] So add some fiber-rich foods—including fruits, most vegetables, oats, rice bran, brown rice, oatmeal, whole wheat products, nuts, and seeds—to your diet along with eight glasses of water daily and give that excess estrogen a flush (no pun intended) right out of your system.

Dr. Lark points out other benefits of whole wheat foods. For example, they are also rich in protein when combined with peas and beans. Plus, grains are high in magnesium, a mineral that relieves menstrual cramps by reducing muscle tension. In addition, the high calcium content in grains also eases muscle contraction, and the potassium content serves as a diuretic and reduces bloating.

But the effects of whole grains aren't all good. If you have severe fibroid symptoms, you may need to eliminate wheat altogether. One reason is that whole wheat contains gluten, a protein that can cause an allergic reaction in many women and is difficult to digest. Further, Lark has seen symptoms such as depression, tiredness, bloating, cramping, diarrhea, and constipation worsen after wheat intake in women that have fibroids or endometriosis along with PMS (premenstrual syndrome). "You may want to try a wheat-free diet to see if you feel better once wheat is eliminated. Also eliminate barley and rye, since they contain gluten as well," Lark asserts. Instead, "substitute buckwheat, rice, and millet."

LEGUMES

Legumes include edible beans, peas, and related pod-bearing plants. Boiled soybeans and soybean products such as tofu, tempeh, soy pasta, soy cheese, and soy yogurt help regulate estrogen production and may spell relief for fibroid sufferers. According to Lark, soy foods "help to reduce bleeding problems in premenopausal women with fibroid tumors." In addition, legumes such as chickpeas, lentils, kidney beans, black beans, pinto beans, soybeans, and lima beans are good sources of iron, copper, and zinc, which are essential to women suffering from anemia. Legumes are also great sources of protein and can be particularly valuable for vegetarians who require meat substitutes. And your body will just love the high levels of vitamin B_6 and vitamin B complex, because these agents help reduce estrogen levels, prevent cramps and tiredness, and promote a healthy functioning liver.

Legumes can also aid in lowering cholesterol and regulating bowel movements. Sometimes that benefit can be accompanied by intestinal gas. To reduce the gas, try adding a digestive enzyme such as powdered ginger or baking soda to your pot while your legumes are cooking. And eat smaller portions. That way you can enjoy the benefit of beans without the uncomfortable aftereffects.

Speaking of Gas

Increasing your intake of grains and bran can be a bloating experience from the excess gas these foods can cause. The same could be said for beans and cruciferous vegetables such as cabbage. But you can avoid the gas buildup by eating these foods in small quantities and by gradually increasing the frequency. In the book *Good Health for*

African Americans (Crown, 1994), author Barbara M. Dixon, R.D., L.D.N., suggests that you *"begin gradually, several times a week, and build to several times a day."* Here are some other suggestions:

- Boil dried beans for two minutes, turn off the heat, and let them sit for an hour. Then pour off the water and cook them as usual using fresh water.
- Increase your intake of yogurt and other fermented foods. The "friendly" bacteria (acidophilus) that they contain aids in the digestion of gassy foods.
- Chew your food completely and eat slowly.
- Refrain from eating when you're feeling tense or upset.
- Avoid overeating.
- Eat small portions.
- Avoid fluid intake while eating.
- Exercise.
- Maintain regular bowel movements.
- Avoid carbonated drinks.
- Nix activities that lead to gas buildup such as gum chewing, sucking on hard candy or straws, drinking large quantities of liquids, and smoking.
- Wild yam relaxes muscular fibers and soothes nerves in the uterus. It also alleviates gas and intestinal irritations.

Go to your nearest health store for these:

- Tincture—15 drops five to seven times daily.
- Herb tea—three to four cups daily.
- Fennel seed—if you find the wild yam doesn't work, drink this brew as needed.

Sources: Dr. Yvonne Paris-Fergerson (Doctorate of Naturopathy); Barbara M. Dixon, R.D., L.D.N., *Good Health for African Americans.*

VEGETABLES

Adding vegetables to your diet can help relieve a number of your fibroid complaints. If you're wondering which ones to tackle first, think green, yellow, and red, as pointed out by Johanna Skilling, author of

Fibroids: The Complete Guide to Taking Charge of Your Physical, Emotional, and Sexual Well-Being (Marlowe & Company, 2000). For example, beta-carotene-filled vegetables such as butternut squash, yams, kale, spinach, and carrots defend against free radicals, molecules that can spark cell abnormalities such as the ones in fibroids. Red tomatoes do an even better job of tackling free radicals.

Green vegetables such as kale, broccoli, cabbage, and arugula combat estrogen by halting the production of the cells that respond to estrogen and transforming estradiol (a more potent form of estrogen) into the milder estrone.

You can rely on vegetables such as Swiss chard, broccoli, spinach, potatoes, sweet potatoes, kale, green peas, green beans, mustard greens, and beet greens as a major source of magnesium, potassium, and calcium. These minerals aid in alleviating cramps and soothing emotions. In addition, these vegetables are also high in iron, a mineral that can help relieve cramping and bleeding.

Load up on potatoes, tomatoes, parsley, peppers, cauliflower, brussels sprouts, and kale for a hefty helping of vitamin C. These capillary strengtheners help reduce excessive bleeding and promote the healing of scars and wounds. Vitamin C–rich vegetables also assist in the production of the adrenal hormone, an agent that helps the body deal with stress.

FRUITS

Trade in the junk food for some healthier fruity snacks. Fruits are loaded with vitamin C, so they can reduce blood flow during heavy periods as well as facilitate blood circulation. Although nearly all fruits are great sources of vitamin C, melons, grapefruits, oranges, and berries are best. You'll also get a healthy helping of bioflavonoids, another capillary-strengthening source that puts the brakes on excessive menstrual bleeding and manages the production of estrogen.

Fruits have loads of other benefits as well. Certain ones—oranges, blackberries, raisins, bananas, and dried figs—are great sources of calcium and magnesium, so load up. If you're suffering from fatigue or bloating, you may get relief by eating potassium-heavy fruits such as bananas, figs, and raisins—although you can get potassium from any fruit.

In addition, the high fiber that fruits contain can remedy a host of other fibroid-related complaints such as digestive problems, constipation, cramping, and menstrual discomfort.

Since fruits offer a wealth of fibroid-fighting agents, you might be tempted to stock up on fruit juice as well. That's not a good idea according to Lark. She says, "Fruit juice does not contain the bulk or fiber of the whole fruit. As a result, it acts more like table sugar and can dramatically destabilize your blood sugar level when used in excess. . . . Less is better. If you want fruit juice, mix it half-and-half with water."

SEEDS, NUTS

Seeds and nuts provide two essential fatty acids—linoleic acid and linolenic acid. This twosome helps your body produce prostaglandin, the hormone that relaxes the muscles and tackles inflammation and cramping. These foods contain vitamin E and B-complex vitamins—two agents that help to alleviate cramps and regulate hormones. In addition, minerals such as calcium, potassium, and magnesium are also found in seeds and nuts.

Which ones should you eat? For both fatty acids, try raw flax and pumpkin seeds. To get linoleic acid alone, snack on sesame and sunflower seeds. The nuts and seeds that are highest on the nutrition scale are almonds, sesame seeds, pecans, pistachios, and sunflower seeds. For the greatest benefits, eat them raw, unsalted, and keep them away from light, oxygen, and heat. Crack them yourself or at the very least refrigerate shelled nuts so they won't spoil. Sprinkle them over salads, casseroles, or other dishes as a garnish. Or, munch on them as a light snack. Just use them sparingly, because nuts and seeds "are very high in calories," cautions Lark.

OILS

Stick to small amounts of vegetable oils when cooking. Vitamin E based oils, such as corn oil, help alleviate moodiness, tiredness, and cramping. Vitamin E also aids in balancing hormones, including estrogen. Olive and canola oils are also good for cooking.

For seasoning vegetables, flavoring rice, or spicing up other dishes, try flax oil. You can also use it as a substitute for butter. Just be aware that flax oil isn't for cooking because it's sensitive to heat, oxygen, and light. It's also extremely perishable. So cook your food first and then add flax oil. Also, keep all oils tightly sealed and refrigerated; don't keep them in a Crisco can on the stove because they'll spoil.

SUGGESTIONS FOR REDESIGNING YOUR DIET

Eating an assortment of vegetables, fruits, and herbs can help you attain a supreme womb, according to Queen Afua. The types of vegetables you should eat include celery, cucumber, parsnip, and other greens. For fruits consider honeydew melons, papaya, mango, and coconut water.

Brother Paur Septah, teacher of wood-carving meditations and nutritional food preparer, claims that whipping up natural food dishes isn't any different from traditional cooking. In fact, it's easier. "People don't realize that seasoning is the only thing that makes meat tasty; if you use some of the same seasonings you use on meat on natural foods or meat substitutes, you'll get the same effect," he insists.

Are you ready to alter your eating habits for better health? Here are some suggestions:

Breakfast

Say goodbye to early morning cereal, bagels, and muffins. Instead, start your day off with fresh fruit and squeezed juices. According to Queen Afua, fruits in the berry family such as cranberries are good for detoxing the womb and bloodstream. You can also eat one to three pieces of fruit such as an apple or pear. Just stay away from bananas during the first month of changing your diet because bananas (especially if they're not ripe) cause gas, bloating, or constipation. "You should have something light, because you're coming from a place of light in the morning," advises Brother Septah. Try the fruity combinations on page 141.

Mind your vitamins and minerals for good health			
Foods naturopaths say you should avoid	Reason	Sources	Exceptions
Dairy products	Causes women to produce higher levels of estrogen and prostaglandin (the cramp-producing hormone). The bovine growth hormone (BGH) given to cows to promote milk pro-duction also produces an insulinlike growth factor-1 hormone, which plays a role in the development of fibroids as well as breast and prostate cancer.	Cow's milk, ice cream, shakes, and butter	Cheese, nonfat yogurt, and milk products be-cause they don't have the prostaglandin-producing agent arachidonic acid.[6]
Meat and poultry	Many animals are treated with anabolic steroids that may have the same effect on women as estrogen.	Beef, pork, deer, lamb, chicken, turkey, and ham	If you must eat meat, try skinless poultry or lean meat. Broil or grill meat and discard remaining fat. Stick to free-range or organically raised meat.
Fats	Saturated fats, which come from animal products. Fat can increase your cholesterol and transform into estrogen. Plus, poly-unsaturated and saturated fats can	Meats, pizza, ice cream, cheese, fried foods, tacos, butter, coconut, cottonseed oils, vegetable shortening, store-baked goods, prepackaged snacks, and other convenience items	Omega-3 fatty acids found in fish such as salmon, herring, bluefish swordfish, mackerel, tuna, and rainbow trout. Also found in wild game, rabbit, flaxseeds, fish oil, walnut oil, wal-nuts, and canola oil.

Foods	Reason	Sources	Exceptions
	convert into "free radicals" which can weaken your immune system.		
Sodium	Can cause high blood pressure (hypertension). Can help people with high blood pressure better control their condition.	Anchovies, cheese, bacon, baking powder, baking soda, catsup, bouillon cubes, cocoa mix, chili sauce, MSG (monosodium glutamate), mustard, green olives, pickles, salad dressing, pizza, barbecue sauce, soy sauce, seasoned salt, table salt, canned vegetables, Worcestershire sauce, teriyaki sauce, sauerkraut, potato chips, salted crackers, nuts, pretzels, popcorn	
Alcohol	Bad for the liver.	Beer, wine, champagne, and some mixed drinks	
Sugar	Sugar raises your insulin level.	Candy, cookies, soda, fruit drinks, white flour products, sweet tea or coffee	
Caffeine	Affects the way your liver functions and its ability to process estrogen. Consuming coffee or tea after meals can reduce the amount of iron your body absorbs.	Coffee, tea, chocolate	Herbal teas
Junk food	High in fat	Potato chips, caffeine, chocolate, soft drinks, fruit juices, fast foods	None

Sound Substitutes		
Substance	*Substitute*	*Comments*
Dairy products	Soy products Soft tofu Soy cheese for cooking Rice, soy, nut or grain milk Nondairy vegetarian butter and cheese substitutes	Try tofu and soy-made yogurt, milk, and ice-cream products. Rice cheese if you are soy intolerant. If you must have animal products, use small amounts of goat's or sheep's milk.
Meat and poultry	Fish Vegetarian-based substitutes	Particularly tuna and salmon. Increase intake of grains, raw seeds, nuts, and beans.
Fats	Olive oil and canola oil	
Sugar	Honey Maple syrup Add extra fruits or nuts in pastries	When substituting these sweeteners for sugar, reduce the liquid content of the recipe by $1/4$ cup. For recipes using solid substances, add 3 to 5 tablespoons for every $3/4$ cup of sweetener. You cannot cook with honey; use as a sweetener for herbal teas.
Table salt	Morton's salt substitute Kelp or Nori (for salads, vegetables, or grains) Low-salt soy sauce Bragg's amino acid (use in small amounts)	Try powdered seaweed. Consider using herbs on meats and vegetables because the flavors are more subtle. Try natural flavorings such as allspice, bay leaf, basil, chives, cinnamon, dry cocoa, cloves, cranberries, fresh ginger, mace, marjoram, mint, dry mustard, fresh onion, parsley, paprika, rosemary, Tabasco, tarragon, thyme, fresh tomato, vinegar, vanilla
Wheat flour	Whole grain non-wheat flour	Try rice flour for pastries, cakes, and cookies. Use barley flour for pie crusts. These substitutes are high in fiber and nutrients such as vitamin B complex and other minerals.
Alcohol	Nonalcoholic or low-alcoholic products, water	Use these substitutes for marinades and sauces that require alcohol for flavoring.

Substance	Substitute	Comments
Caffeine	Coffee substitutes such as Pero, Postum, and Caffix Decaffeinated coffee and teas Herb tea (e.g., ginger tea)	Try grain-based coffee substitutes.

Substitutes for Common High-Stress Ingredients	
¾ cup sugar	½ cup honey (remember, you cannot cook with honey because it will become toxic) ¼ cup molasses ½ cup maple syrup ½ ounce barley malt 1 cup apple butter 2 cups apple juice
1 cup milk	1 cup soy, potato, nut, or grain milk
1 tablespoon butter	1 tablespoon flax oil (must be used raw and unheated)
½ teaspoon salt	1 tablespoon miso ½ teaspoon potassium chloride salt substitute ½ teaspoon Mrs. Dash, Spike ½ teaspoon herbs (basil, tarragon, oregano, etc.)
1 square chocolate	¾ tablespoon powdered carob
1 tablespoon coffee	1 tablespoon decaffeinated coffee 1 tablespoon Pero, Postum, Caffix, or other grain-based coffee substitutes
4 ounces wine	4 ounces light wine
8 ounces beer	8 ounces near beer
1 cup white flour	1 cup barley flour (for pie crusts) 1 cup rice flour (for cookies, cakes, breads)

FUN FRUIT BREAKFAST MIXTURES

Option #1

Cut up an apple or pear (or use both).

Drop in ½ to 1 cup of strawberries. Enjoy.

Option #2

½ cup of mixed strawberries or raspberries.

Option #3

Juice fresh grapefruit, pineapple, orange, apple, or unsweetened cranberry until you get 4 ounces.

Then add 4 ounces of distilled or purified water.

Lunch

"Your heaviest meal should be consumed during lunchtime," states Brother Septah. Aside from breakfast and dessert, all of your meals should consist of a large raw green salad as the base. Then add other foods around it for variety. Use the salad recipe for lunch and dinner.

BASIC SALAD

Chop and mix the following ingredients:

1 large romaine lettuce leaf chopped up
1 large watercress leaf
1 sprig parsley
1 cucumber
1 avocado
1 package seaweed (crush it and sprinkle over salad)

DRESSING:

Place these items in a blender for mixing:

1 package chopped tofu
2 cloves garlic
1 teaspoon Spike
4 to 5 teaspoons Bragg's Liquid Amino
½ medium onion
2 teaspoons olive oil

OR

Same recipe above; just leave out the tofu

Lunch

Option #1

Season tufu and scamble it (as you would an egg) and add on salad.

Option #2
SLAMMIN JAMMIN LAMMIN HAMMIN

2 cups vegetarian ham "made from soy products"
2 cups vegetarian lamb* "made from soy products"
1 tablespoon Bragg's Liquid Amino
Dice or puree and add the following:
1 red pepper
1 green pepper
1 onion
2 cloves garlic
4 scotch bonnet peppers (sweet)
¼ teaspoon basil
¼ teaspoon cayenne pepper
½ teaspoon Spike
Smidgen olive oil
1 cup distilled or purified water
Cook down until it speaks to you.

*The lamb, as do some other vegetarian meats, comes dry. Before you cook with it, soak it in boiling water for about an hour.

Dinner

Have another salad for dinner. But for spice add grain such as couscous, bulgur wheat (unless you're allergic), or tabouli.

Girlfriend, I know what you're thinking. This change is pretty drastic. Well, it's going to take a drastic change to get some drastic results. And isn't that the point?

Of course, there really are no guarantees here. Many doctors feel there is absolutely no relationship between food intake and fibroids. I find that hard to believe but decide for yourself. In the meantime, try Barbara Dixon's healthier soul food delights.

Healthier Substitutes for Your Favorite Soul Food
(Remember to use the sound substitutes.)

Southern Oven Fried Chicken

1 free-range chicken (2½ to 3 pounds)
—remove and discard the skin
¼ teaspoon Mrs. Dash or Spike
½ teaspoon garlic powder
½ teaspoon curry powder
¼ teaspoon ground cumin
¼ teaspoon paprika
¼ teaspoon ground red pepper
(optional)

¼ teaspoon ground black pepper
½ cup of all-purpose flour
¼ cup yellow cornmeal
½ cup low-fat or nonfat buttermilk
1 tablespoon low-sodium
Worcestershire sauce
1 tablespoon mustard
Nonstick butter-flavored vegetable spray

Preheat oven to 350° Fahrenheit. Divide chicken into six to eight serving-size segments. Remove the bone from breast. Save the wings, back, and bones for stock. Combine and mix the Mrs. Dash/Spike, garlic powder, curry powder, cumin, paprika, red pepper, and black pepper in a small bowl. Put ½ teaspoon of the mixture to the side and use the remaining substance to season the chicken.

In a shallow baking dish, mix the cornmeal, flour, and the seasoning that you saved. Put to the side.

Next beat together the Worcestershire sauce, milk, and mustard in a medium size bowl. Coat each piece of chicken with this substance, then roll into the flour mix. Spray a large baking sheet with the cooking spray and arrange the chicken pieces neatly on it. Then spray each piece of chicken with the cooking spray to help it retain moisture. Finally, bake for 30 minutes until the chicken is golden brown, tender, and crisp.

Source: *Good Health for African Americans* (Crown, 1994, $14).

Sesame Oven Fried Fish

1 pound catfish or other fillet
(fresh or frozen)
¼ cup skim milk
½ cup fine dry bread crumbs

½ cup yellow cornmeal
1 tablespoon toasted sesame seeds
1 tablespoon Mrs. Dash seasoning
¼ teaspoon dry mustard

Oven should be preheated to 450° Fahrenheit. If you use frozen fish, thaw it out. Next, dip fish in milk and then coat with bread crumbs. Spray cooking sheet with vegetable spray and place the fish neatly on it. Bake until fish is golden brown. For each 2-inch thickness of fish, allow 4 to 6 minutes of cooking time.

Delectable Desserts

Rice Pudding Supreme

⅓ cup raw short-grain brown rice
1 ¼ cups nonfat milk
½ cup instant powdered nonfat milk
½ cup frozen apple juice concentrate
2 tablespoons pure vanilla extract
4 egg whites, beaten until foamy

1 ripe banana pureed
⅔ cup muscat raisins, plumped (place in covered bowl with hot water for 15 minutes)
1 teaspoon ground cinnamon
freshly ground nutmeg
1 cup Grape-Nuts cereal

Cook rice in 1 cup boiling water for 25 minutes and then set aside. Mix together nonfat and powdered milk and heat until boiling. Reduce heat. Add the apple juice concentrate, egg whites, vanilla, pureed banana, and blend well.

Put cooked rice in a 1-quart ovenproof casserole. Add raisins and pour on the milk mixture. Next sprinkle cinnamon, ground nutmeg, and Grape-Nuts.

Place the casserole in a baking dish with 1 inch hot water and bake for 45 to 50 minutes. Test it by inserting a sharp knife in it and pulling it out. When it comes out clean, the custard is done.

MAINTAINING A FOOD DIARY

In the book *Good Health for African Americans* (Crown, 1994, $14), author Barbara M. Dixon, R.D., L.D.N., suggests that maintaining a food diary will help you stay motivated to track and improve your eating habits. You can start by using a clean white piece of paper kept in a three-ring binder or spiral notebook. Or you can go high-tech and develop a chart on your computer or Palm Pilot. Next, record your start date, age, and vital statistics—measurements for your height, weight, bust, waist, hips, thighs, and upper arms—as they are on the date that you begin. Then start recording ALL of the beverages and food that you consume (if you're not sure of the full ingredients in lasagna, take your best guess), the date, where you ate it (restaurant, home, or work, for example), and what emotions you were feeling when you ate it. This will help you identify trends and develop strategies to change bad habits. For example, if you notice you're consuming more fatty foods when you eat at work during late nights or when you're depressed, maybe you should start bringing healthier snacks to work or start talking out your problems when you're depressed so you won't eat as much.

Later, add another column so you can record the amount of calories you're ingesting during each meal; you can find this information out by reading the labels on the foods you consume and purchasing a calorie counter in your local bookstore. There are also computer programs that calculate the amount of calories you're getting from carbohydrates, fat, and protein. But you can do this yourself by reading the label and doing the following computations:

- For each gram of carbohydrates and protein multiply each number by 4.
- For each gram of fat multiply that number by 9.

The key is to record everything, even the three fries that you scooped up from your friend's lunch—calories can add up. According to Dixon, "The purpose of the food diary is not to launch a guilt trip but to determine what you *really* eat, and how much, on a daily basis. *You don't need to show your diary to anyone.*"

Dr. Susan Love, author of *Dr. Susan Love's Hormone Book: Making Informed Choices About Menopause,* agrees. In her book, she says that maintaining a food diary is part of the work that needs to be done to transition from the ever-popular high-fat, low-fiber diet to a more healthy diet. "When you look at your own diary after a week and see everything you've been consuming, you're likely to be surprised—and maybe even appalled," she says.

Use the chart below as a guide. Feel free to add more columns to suit your specific needs. Just be honest. "Some experts say that just by keeping an *honest* food diary, you can lose a pound a week," adds Dixon. More importantly, you'll be a few steps closer to a healthier you. Don't forget to drink at least eight cups of water daily. Let the diary begin . . .

Sample Food Diary

Date	Time of day (incl. A.M. or P.M.)	Breakfast	Lunch	Dinner	Other Meals	Where did I eat this meal?	What emotion was I feeling when I ate?	How hungry am I? (1 = not hungry at all, 5 = extremely hungry)

Recommended Daily Allowance

Fat	30% or less of your total calories
Protein	Two or three servings* per day from meats or beans

*1 serving = 8 ounces

Fat Busters

Reduce the fat in your diet.[7]
- Decrease your intake of poultry and meat to one serving per week. (A serving is 3 ounces or about the size of a deck of cards.)
- Trim the fat or skin off of red meat or poultry and you'll cut your calories in half.
- Choose leaner meats over high-fat ones.
- Substitute ground turkey or chicken for ground beef.
- Avoid fast foods or processed meats.
- Substitute fresh fruit or applesauce for sugar when cooking. Try to reduce the amount of sugar you typically add to recipes by 80 percent.
- Use diet salad dressings. Also try diet salad dressing as a marinade over meats.
- Choose low-fat or no-fat dairy items. (If you're still eating dairy products.)

8 Fibroid Shape-up

Exercise Your Way to Relief

A lot of working women sit for long periods of time, go home and go to bed, and never really get a chance to do any stretching or exercise. As a result, the womb area becomes very blocked with oxygen and blood flow and this is the breeding ground for disease.

Exercise helps to increase blood flow and oxygen into your body and cells. That's important because this helps your cells function at optimal levels.

My advice to everyone is to really take health and wellness into your own hands. Become knowledgeable about your body and what goes on with it. Stay as close to nature as much as possible. And know that while synthetic medication and surgery may help alleviate illness and disease, you should use it as a last resort instead of a first option. Disease only returns when you don't address the root of the problem.

—Empress Zuleika Bes Sekhemet Maat, Age 31
Womb Dance Instructor

Sis, if fibroids have got you down, maybe it's time for you to start whipping those myomas into shape by stepping up your exercise program—or starting one if you don't already have one. Why? Exercise does wonders for your overall health and may relieve some of your fibroid symptoms as well. According to the National Institutes of Health, athletic women appear to have fewer fibroids than their less active counterparts. Apparently fibroids aren't fond of a good workout. Aside from possibly keeping your fibroids at bay or at least keeping them in check, a solid exercise program will help eliminate excess estrogen by reducing your cholesterol, fat content, and insulin levels. Staying active also increases your blood and oxygen circulation, soothes your muscles, and calms menstrual symptoms. In addition, exercise boosts energy, reduces stress, and alleviates cramps. Further, exercise helps your body release endorphins, painkilling chemicals that are manufactured by your brain. And aerobics can help to balance the autonomic nervous system;

this can reduce anxiety and calm your mood. All of these benefits should help you better manage your fibroids. But don't just take my word for it; get to stepping.

Go running, walking, swimming, dancing, or bike riding to start enjoying the healthy benefits of an active lifestyle. If you're a fibroid sufferer who has menstrual cramps or lower back pain, Dr. Susan Lark suggests stretching and flexibility exercises. She also recommends yoga and breathing exercises for the treatment of back pain, cramps, and lower congestion.

The key is to listen to your body, so don't overdo it. If your fibroids have gotten to the point that exercise is painful or overly strenuous, then you may have to wait until you're able to gain control over your condition before starting a workout. In any case, go to your doctor for a full examination to ensure that you're in good physical condition prior to starting any exercise program. The bottom line is that you don't have to use your fibroids as an excuse for not exercising. This chapter will provide some ideas to help you increase your physical activity as well as show you how to incorporate it into your lifestyle.

WHY YOU DON'T EXERCISE

Although there are a number of black women who do work out, many of us don't work out at all. We're less likely to exercise than black men and white women.[1] In fact, a 1992 Centers for Disease Control and Prevention survey reported that 43 percent of African American women (ages eighteen or older) didn't participate in "leisure-time physical activity." Research indicates that African Americans view exercise as stressful, and the relationship between good health and exercise has never been fully emphasized in our community. Yet our sedentary lifestyle is killing us. In addition, the high prevalence of fibroids in African American women may be partially explained by their tendency to be overweight resulting from lack of exercise.

But you have good reasons for not exercising—right? I know all of the excuses and have used a few myself a time or two. In the book *Body & Soul: The Black Women's Guide to Physical Health and Emotional Well-Being* (HarperPerennial, $22), author Linda Villarosa points out some of the reasons that black women use to explain why they don't exercise. Even though these excuses may *sound* like good reasons for not giving your body the workout it deserves, let's look at why these excuses and others really don't hold up.

"I don't have enough time to exercise." Says who? The latest research shows that you can gain enormous benefits from relatively modest exercise. A twenty-minute stroll, for example, can significantly decrease your cholesterol and blood pressure. It can also lower your risk of high blood pressure, heart attack, and stroke.[2] Even if you participate in physical activity just one day a week, you'll significantly reduce your risk of diabetes. Also any exercising you do adds up. So start by taking three brisk walks of ten minutes each every day. Then add other activities to your program.

"I don't like to exercise." I bet there are some activities that you like doing or may be participating in already. Remember, you don't have to run, jog, bicycle ride, or go to the gym for a workout. In the book *Like a Natural Woman*, author Ziba Kashef offers some interesting exercise alternatives, including Eastern practices such as yoga, chi kung, and tai chi as well as culturally centered activities such as capoeira and African dance. You can also play Ping-Pong, garden, shovel snow, roller-skate, or increase play with your kids. "If you can't find physical activities you enjoy, recall the ones you liked years ago," writes Michael Castleman in his book *Nature's Cures: From Acupressure & Aromatherapy to Walking & Yoga, the Ultimate Guide to the Best Scientifically Proven, Drug-Free Healing Methods* (Bantam, $6.99). "Chances are you'll still enjoy them."

"I don't know how." Baloney. Start by looking at the physical activities you're already participating in such as cooking, housework, shopping, and child care. Look for ways to participate in those chores more briskly and bend and stretch while you're cooking or cleaning. Also, park your car further from your destinations so you can do more walking. Then search the Internet and other publications, such as *Heart & Soul*, for more ideas. *Black Enterprise* magazine, for example, ran an article entitled "Office-Worthy Workout" (November 1999) that featured a series of exercises that can be performed right at your desk.

"I'm too overweight to start exercising now." There's no better time than the present. Don't be embarrassed about your weight. Instead, use it as motivation for you to whip yourself into shape. People will be inspired by you and appreciate your efforts to take steps toward improved health. Plus, you'll enjoy the added flexibility, stamina, and strength that exercise promotes. And you'll feel better about yourself because you're finally taking responsibility for your own happiness and well-being.

"I'm too tired." Aren't we all? Still, exercise will help you feel less tired overall because physical activity sharpens mental alertness. In addition, physical activity stimulates the brain's production of painkilling endorphins and neurotransmitters, chemicals that elevate mood and reduce fatigue. Further, exercise is also associated with the energy boost known as a "runner's high." So start energizing yourself with a good exercise program.

"I don't have access to workout facilities." You don't need them. Vigorous housework is good exercise. Also, you can rent a number of exercise tapes at your neighborhood video store. And you can increase your walking and running on your way to work or to the mall.

"I don't have a babysitter." Children make great exercise partners. Try exercising together so they get into the habit of exercising at an early age. If they're too small, consider exercising before they awake or after they go to bed.

"I don't see any progress." Maybe it's because you're not keeping track of it. Record your daily exercise habits as well as the time associated with each activity. Then periodically review your records. For example, look at how long it took for you to walk a mile six months ago and how long it takes you today. You should see a significant difference if you've been exercising consistently. Also, focus on the positive. Celebrate all of the little achievements along the way—not by taking a break from exercise, of course.

"I can't stick with it." Unfortunately, that's a common complaint. About 50 percent of people who start exercising throw in the towel after six months. There are a couple of ways to increase your chances of success. First, start slowly. Get into an exercise program gradually; if you take on too much too soon, you'll become discouraged. Next, part-

ner up with someone who loves to exercise so their enthusiasm will rub off on you. And don't overdo it. Experts say you should be able to hold a conversation with someone while you're exercising. If you find yourself breathless, your workout is too vigorous. The thing to remember is that once you stop exercising, "the benefits diminish within just a couple of weeks and completely disappear within a few months," writes Kashef. Still, if you do stop exercising, she also advises that you "forgive yourself and start again. It's not about rules, but fun and feeling good."

"I don't have time to see my physician." There's nothing more important than your good health, so make the time. That said, you probably don't have to see a physician right away if you're only starting a modest exercise program and don't have any specific health problems. But definitely do consult your physician prior to participating in any exercise if you're over fifty, are pregnant, or have a family or personal history of asthma, diabetes, heart disease, hypertension, varicose veins, or any other medical condition.

"Exercise hurts." If that's the case, then you're probably overdoing it. Your exercise program should not be causing sharp pain; if it is, you should stop doing it. If you're a new exerciser (especially if you're out of shape), you'll probably feel soreness for twelve to forty-eight hours after the activity. Once the aches subside, you can resume your exercise program. As time goes on, the soreness will stop unless you increase the length or intensity of your workout.

Are you ready to put those excuses away now? If so, start making exercise a daily part of your routine. You'll look better and feel better. Most of all, you'll become an active participant in shaping a better you.

Exercise Benefits Beyond Fibroid Management

Helps manage weight.
Boosts sexual responsiveness.
Reduces risk of heart disease and stroke.
Lowers cholesterol.
Aids in preserving bones.
Builds flexibility, stamina, and strength.
Enhances reaction time.
Improves memory.

Boosts immune system.
May prevent insomnia.
Relieves arthritis.
Instills greater self-confidence.
Elevates mood.
Fights disease.
Relieves depression and stress.
Aids in reproductive problems.

GET STARTED, GIRL

Becoming physically fit requires that you beef up three areas—flexibility, strength, and stamina—through your exercise program. To increase your flexibility, participate in stretching and yoga exercises. As you become more flexible, you won't strain or pull a muscle when you reach for things or stoop. For more strength, do a nonstop twenty-to-thirty-minute weight-training workout. This will help you burn calories, shed fat, and build up muscle for a leaner, trimmer look. In addition, you can build stamina by participating in an aerobic activity such as running, brisk walking, basketball, skating, or any vigorous activity for twenty to thirty minutes at least three times a week.

If you're ready to map out a program that's right for your age, body type, health condition, and goals, consult a certified personal fitness trainer and conduct your research by referring to the Internet, exercise tapes, and various publications. Here are some additional tips:

- Start slowly. You should be able to carry on a conversation. If you're a beginner, for example, walk fast enough to increase your heart rate but not to pant.
- Wear the proper shoes when you're doing aerobics, preferably a pair with support and lots of cushion.
- Warm up with ten minutes of stretching prior to participating in vigorous exercise. Then end your exercise program with another five to ten minutes of stretching to cool down.
- Set aside adequate exercise time, approximately thirty minutes.
- Wear comfortable clothes and exercise without socks for freedom of movement and to avoid slipping.

- Evacuate your bowels or bladder prior to exercising and wait two hours after eating before you work out.
- Figure out your "target heart zone." Subtract your age from 220 to get your maximum heart rate (MHR). Then multiply that result by .65 and then multiply the same MHR by .80. The two numbers give you the target heart zone range.
- Take your pulse while you're exercising. Put two fingers (not your thumb) on the big artery on the side of your neck or the artery in your wrist, then count the beats for fifteen seconds and multiply the result by 4. It should be in your target heart zone.
- Increase the intensity, duration, and frequency of your exercise activity.
- Set goals for each activity. Then reward yourself once you achieve your goal.
- Drink lots of water throughout your workout to cool your body and replenish lost fluid.
- Progress slowly through your exercises because this promotes flexibility and prevents injury.
- For safer exercises, consider biking, swimming, and walking.
- Pay attention to your body. Pain is a signal that something is wrong, so discontinue any hurtful activity.
- Purchase the right equipment for your workout, including a sports bra, shoes, and other equipment.

Exercise Daily

Take a walk.
Choose the stairs over the elevator.
Wear walking shoes to work instead of your heels.
Use a backpack for carrying things so you'll free up your hands.
Park further away from your destinations.
Avoid breakfast, lunch, or dinner meetings.
Walk your dog or someone else's pooch.
Exercise during your short breaks.
Choose a live visit over a telephone call.
Exercise while chatting on the telephone.
Do more household chores such as mowing the lawn, gardening, shoveling snow, or cleaning out the garage or attic.
Participate in more physical activity with your kids.

NEED SOME FIBROID-RELIEVING EXERCISE IDEAS?

In her book *Sacred Woman: A Guide to Healing the Feminine Body, Mind, and Spirit* (Ballantine, $28), Queen Afua suggests that women have a dialogue with their womb through exercise. Her "Dance of the Womb" features a series of twenty-five rhythmic movements that are designed to create a well-rounded, vibrant, healthy uterus. It takes approximately thirty to sixty minutes to complete this regimen, but you can do the movements for as long as you like. Here are other ideas:

Inhale, Exhale

Would you believe that the way you breathe can affect your fibroid symptoms? According to Dr. Susan Lark, practicing therapeutic breathing exercises can diminish anxiety, relax muscles, minimize pain, and create a feeling of peace. Here are some techniques that may work for you:

Breath Massage for Stress Relief
While lying flat on your back, take air through your nose allowing it to flow down to your abdomen. As you're inhaling, envision yourself being filled with positive energy and allow your abdomen to fully expand. Now exhale and become intimately aware of each of the air molecules that leave your body. Do you feel better? Good; try this method as often as you like.

A Grounded Breath for Centeredness
As you sit upright in a chair, place both feet slightly apart on the floor. Inhale through your nose allowing your abdomen to fill completely. Hold it. Now imagine there are three long cords, one running from your rear end and the other two running from your feet. All of the cords meet at the center of the earth. Focus on that point until you need to release the air.

A Color-Filled Breath for Energy
Use this exercise for strength and healing. You can use various colors such as red, gold, or blue. We'll use red here. For this technique, you can sit or lie down on your back. Now, as you take a deep breath, imagine that the world beneath you is red. Next allow your energy center on the bottom of your feet to open up, and draw in this color up through your legs and then your womb. Visualize your uterus filling up

with red light. Now, as you exhale, allow the red light to wash away or dissolve your fibroids. As the color disappears, you can envision your fibroids evaporating as well. This approach should be done five times consecutively.

GIVE STRESS A REST

African American women are more stressed out than their white counterparts, so it's no wonder that their uteruses are bombarded with fibroids—a condition that appears to be stress-related. But you don't have to ask researchers whether stress impacts fibroids; just ask the women who suffer from them. In a survey conducted by Dr. Ann Chopelas, 44 percent of the women respondents could link specific periods of significant stress with their fibroid growth. In the same survey, 27 percent of respondents reported that simply having fibroids elevated their stress levels.

How does stress affect your fibroids? Stress causes us to tense various parts of the body. It may trigger you to subconsciously contract your pelvic muscles, which can cut off the supply of nutrients to your organs and contract the blood flow to the pelvis. In response, the oxygen level in those areas drops and that can produce lactic acid, which can trigger discomfort and cramping and prevent toxins from being properly expelled from the body.

Overall, there are theories that suggest how stress can make your fibroids grow and worsen the symptoms associated with them, according to Johanna Skilling. Stress depresses your immune system, which increases the intensity of your symptoms and prevents you from fighting off infection; inspires you to indulge in various types of fibroid-friendly habits like consuming sweets, alcohol, and dairy products; and enables your body to release estrogen-raising toxins in the body. And if that's not enough, just dealing with the troubles that accompany fibroids along with the other issues that black women have to deal with including family life, work, financial challenges, and racism can be especially stressful. In fact, Sir Abdulla Smithford, a naturopathic physician, says, "stress, in my opinion, causes greater damage than anything else in regard to fibroids."

So if you want to get a handle on your fibroids and other daily challenges, try moving from "stress victim to stress victor," advises Dr.

Stress Triggers and Stress Relievers		
Problem	*Stress Signals*	*Solution*
Working too hard	Yelling at coworkers, missing deadlines, being overly agitated, feeling overwhelmed, underperforming	Tell others how you're feeling and ask for help. Learn to delegate. Take breaks during the day and stop skipping lunches. Take a vacation day. Putting distance between you and your work can do wonders.
Overcommitting yourself	Missing obligations. Feeling cheated for denying your own wants. Blaming others because you keep breaking your promises. Excessive lateness. Being overly tired.	Learn to say "No." Also know that you have the right to change your mind if you give people enough time to make other plans or offer a better solution—just don't make this a habit. Also ensure that you schedule enough time for you to realistically complete your obligation.
Disorganized	Lost keys, misplaced paperwork, untidy work area or home, missed buses, or other inconveniences that could have been avoided.	Take a time management course. Consult a professional about better organizing your life. Also learn to put things such as keys, phone books, or other items you use regularly back in their right place.
Financially crunched	Bounced checks, late payment notices, maxed-out credit cards, calls or letters from bill collectors, and a feeling of embarrassment about your financial situation.	Set a budget and stick to it. Avoid impulse purchases. When you go food shopping, purchase only the items on your list. Start taking your lunch to work, and rent movies instead of going to the theater.
Lonely	Depression, jealousy, anger, resentment, and isolation.	Start getting out more. Join a social club, take a class,

Problem	Stress Signals	Solution
		or invite a friend or co-worker to lunch. Host a small mixer at a nearby hangout or your home.
Bad habits	Traffic jams, excessive lateness, poor presentations, inconsiderate gestures, petty arguments, and feeling as if you're always running behind schedule.	Practice better planning. Leave earlier, go to bed earlier, write things down so you won't forget things that are important to others, and treat people as you want to be treated.
Unfulfilling relationships	Poor communication, arguments, unloving exchanges, use of degrading language, and lack of support.	Don't spend any time with people who encourage you to argue, lie, gossip, whine, or wallow in your misery. The majority of your day should be with people who will further your destiny and allow you to further theirs.
Unsupportive environments	Engulfed by gossipers or naysayers. Allowing distractions to keep you from getting as much work done as you planned. Feeling down as soon as you arrive at a particular setting.	Avoid settings that make you feel down. Distance yourself from gossipers, naysayers, or other negative energy.
Overweight	Failing to fit comfortably in your clothes. Responding to an emotional challenge by overeating. Having poor self-esteem.	No matter what size you are, wear clothes that fit. Also wear clothes that showcase your best feature and wear colors that complement your shape and complexion. Start a food journal and cut down on your meals. Hook up with a nutritionist, workout trainer, and physician for guidance.

Grace Cornish, author of *10 Good Choices That Empower Black Women's Lives* (Crown, $21). "Pinpoint the situations that make you feel tense," she says. These could include major lifestyle changes, work challenges, family issues, minor irritations, or a combination of these elements. Then once you identify the problems that "make you feel uneasy, angry, or miserable, you must make adjustments to ease the tension." And that doesn't mean turning to alcohol, smoking, drugs, or other destructive behavior.

HAVE SOME FUN

Exercise and meditation are excellent ways to reduce stress, so incorporate them into your daily living today. Here are some other things you can do to chill out:

Groove to your favorite jam. Turn up the radio, girl, and dance like nobody's watching you. It might feel strange at first, but you'll become the best dance partner you've ever had.

Enjoy some bubbly. No, I'm not talking about alcohol. Submerge yourself in a soothing bubble bath and surround yourself with sweet-smelling candles for the ultimate relaxation. The water should be warm because heat increases your menstrual flow.

If you have a particular fibroid complaint, try Dr. Lark's special brews.

Alkaline Bath for cramps, muscle tension, irritability, insomnia, and anxiety:

- Fill tub with warm water.
- 1 cup sea salt
- 1 cup bicarbonate soda
- Sit for 20 minutes before going to bed.
- Use only once or twice a month.

Hydrogen Peroxide Bath for tense muscles:

- Fill tub with warm water.
- 3 pints 3% peroxide solution

OR

- 6 ounces stronger peroxide solution
- Soak for 30 minutes.

Enjoy a good book. Whether you choose to flip through the pages of your favorite novel or listen to your favorite Bible verses on tape, taking the focus off your fibroids will help you better deal with them.

DON'T WORRY, BE HAPPY AND WORK OUT

The bottom line here is that you can largely impact your fibroids by exercising and managing your stress. You'll look better and feel better—what could be better than that? Dr. Cornish suggests you "get into the happiness habit" by making a list of six things that make you happy so you can meditate on them throughout the day and prior to going to bed for a pleasant sleep. That sounds like a good idea to me. But I'd like you to go a step further. Don't just list things that made you happy throughout the day, think about the things that have made you happy throughout the day and the course of your lifetime. As the song goes, count your many blessings and see what God has done (I know I've abbreviated here but you get the picture). Once you've done that, make a commitment to take better care of yourself. After all, your body is too valuable to waste.

Here's what the Creator has done for me:

I am healthy.

_____

_____

_____

_____

_____

Here's how I'm going to take care of those gifts:

I am going to join a gym on (put in the date) and take at least a 15-minute walk daily.

_____

_____

_____

_____

_____

Here's how I plan to reduce my stress:

_____

_____

_____

_____

_____

9 Techniques of Touch

Acupuncture, Massage Therapy, Reflexology, and Other Bodywork

The premise of Reiki is that based on energy channeling and the promise that God has given us all, we need to heal ourselves. Energy is both negative and positive. And you would have a lot of negative around something that causes you dis-ease, stress, or pain. Instead of just dealing with that pain, we deal with the core issue and begin the practice of positive energy channeling to remove the negativity.

Fibroids are caused by negative energy. Reiki healers address fibroids by channeling energy through the second chakra. By doing this, we don't expect them to grow again and give problems. We believe the development of fibroids is a manifestation of something that hasn't been dealt with. When we start to deal with the negative energy surrounding the fibroids we find that there is a release and a healing.

—Karima, Age 34, Reiki Healer

Do you remember the last time you got a bump or bruise? I bet I can tell you the first thing that you did—rub it. That's because hands, at least to some degree, have the power to heal or ease pain. The process of rubbing, massaging, touching, or adding pressure may provide some relief for your fibroid symptoms as well.

Using techniques of touch to heal is nothing new for us. As Ziba Kashef points out in her book *Like a Natural Woman* (Kensington, $15), our ancestors were among the first to use hands-on therapies for healing. Touch therapy dates back to a time when humans didn't have drugs or medical instruments for remedies—their hands were all they had. Further, the Bible advocates the laying of hands on the sick for recovery. In Mark, chapters 1 and 2, Jesus laid hands on the sick and crippled to heal their bodies. There are various instances throughout our history where touching, holding, hugging, and massaging were used to remedy various ailments.

Present-day practitioners have developed teaching programs and field names for techniques that were once second nature to African Americans. Although traditional healing practices may not fully be able to withstand the criticism of modern-day physicians because the effects of these treatments aren't fully documented or understood, the skepticism has led to further research. This additional research has enabled practitioners to upgrade their techniques and discover new uses for them. In addition, the intense scrutiny that alternative therapy has undergone has caught the attention of many physicians practicing Western medicine. According to Michael Castleman, author of *Nature's Cures: From Acupressure & Aromatherapy to Walking & Yoga, the Ultimate Guide to the Best Scientifically Proven, Drug-Free Healing Methods* (Bantam, $6.99), "Over the last decade, several natural therapies that were once considered alternative have become largely integrated into conventional medicine. Among them are exercise, low-fat diet, massage, meditation, dietary supplements and yoga." Instead of looking at touch therapies as an alternative, try using these remedies to complement the treatment plan prescribed by your physician.

In this chapter, we will look at the various types of bodywork that have been used to treat fibroid symptoms and discuss the results. Further, this section will highlight the wide range of benefits you can achieve by using techniques such as acupuncture, acupressure, aromatherapy, massage therapy, reflexology, Reiki healing, sitz baths, and meditation.

WHAT RESULTS CAN YOU EXPECT FROM TECHNIQUES OF TOUCH?

That's the real question, isn't it? Even though these drug-free approaches sound hip, they make sense only if you're going to get the results you want. The truth is that no one really knows how the use of these nontraditional techniques will impact your condition. As Johanna Skilling points out in her book *Fibroids: The Complete Guide to Taking Charge of Your Physical, Emotional, and Sexual Well-Being* (Marlowe & Company, 2000, $15.95), most alternative therapies seem to offer the promise of relief from fibroid symptoms rather than shrinking the fibroids themselves. Overall, the outcome for these nontraditional therapies is unpredictable because these methods aren't supported by any tests that can generate consistent results.

In many instances natural medicine and Western medicine are at opposite ends of the spectrum. With Western medicine, your physician can tell you with a degree of certainty the results you can expect and when the effect will occur because the treatments he prescribes have been tested by using peer-reviewed studies and control groups that account for variations that could affect results. In addition, Western medicine is regulated by government agencies such as the Food and Drug Administration (FDA), an organization that regulates the drugs and foods that are produced and sold in the United States. Moreover, the results from Western medicine typically happen quick-fast-and-in-a-hurry. For example, you may feel relief from painkillers almost immediately and your symptoms should improve within hours after you have surgery.

Alternative therapies are just that—an alternate way of experiencing healing. The results, if any, are slow; they could take anywhere from a few months to years. Unlike Western medicine, alternative therapies are not regulated by a government agency or widely tested. There is no concrete evidence to demonstrate when they should be used or to support their effectiveness. As Dr. Yvonne Thornton cautions, "When patients go to these [nontraditional practitioners] they are taking their health in their own hands."

Even when natural practitioners do report rave results, the findings aren't consistent and can't be easily duplicated. Improvements are always most prevalent in women in their forties and fifties. This age group would typically experience a shrinkage of fibroids anyway—even without natural remedies—because females are either in the perimenopausal or the postmenopausal stage, when estrogen levels are significantly diminished.

Girlfriend, it's important that you assess natural practitioners with the same critical eye you'd use to check out a conventional physician. Just as you'd comb the Internet and other resources before agreeing to have surgery or taking medication, you should also take a sensible approach when exploring alternative therapy practitioners. That means securing recommendations from people that you know, or at the very least, getting some insight from a national organization that deals with the specialty, such as the Office of Alternate Medicine, Associated Bodywork and Massage Professionals, American Association of Acupuncture and Oriental Medicine (AAAOM), and the Complementary Medical Association. Also, check out the practitioner with the Better Business Bureau in your state to find out if they have any complaints lodged against them. Finally, don't ignore your female intuition. If something doesn't sit quite right with you or if your symptoms seem to be getting worse, don't be afraid to pass on the practitioner.

That said, some women report that their fibroid symptoms respond to alternative healing techniques. In the book *Women's Encyclopedia of Natural Medicine: Alternative Therapies and Integrative Medicine* (Keats, 1999, $24.95), author Tori Hudson, N.D., states that practitioners and patients reported individual case studies indicating that natural therapies can shrink the size of fibroids. These findings were supported by pelvic ultrasound readings, fading symptoms, and reports of complete disappearance of women's fibroids. An article in *Ebony* magazine also found black women who had experienced success by using natural therapies. It stated that "an increasing number of Black women are turning to alternative, or holistic, medicine like nutritional therapy, herbal medicines and even Chinese acupuncture in an effort to find relief from their fibroids. . . . Sisters say they are getting positive results from their unconventional therapy, even claiming that their fibroids shrank."

So what does that mean for you? If your fibroids are small, you may want to try one of the nonsurgical, nonconventional healing approaches. You could be the one to receive a miraculous recovery or your symptoms may diminish. And even if your fibroids don't respond to the treatments, you may still experience a wealth of other benefits that are associated with healing through touch (see sidebar on page 176). Just select an approach that's right for you by reviewing the descriptions of the various touch techniques, their advantages and limitations.

ENERGIZE YOURSELF BY MANAGING YOUR CHAKRAS

According to Eastern cultures, humans have seven energy centers in the body called chakras (see illustration on page 179). They run parallel to the body's neuroendocrine immune system while forming a bond between the physical and energy anatomy. Each chakra relates to a specific organ and is affected by various emotional states. Chakras provide the bridge between the body's hormones, nerves, and emotions.

Women who have fibroids are said to suffer from an imbalance of the second chakra, the energy center associated with the pelvic and reproductive organs. Some physical challenges that emerge are OB/GYN problems such as pain in the pelvic area and lower back, lack of creativity, sexual dysfunction, urinary problems, and appendicitis. These issues typically result from issues surrounding trust, control, blame, or guilt and reveal themselves through problems with sex, money, relationships, fertility, codependency, and people skills. The key here is to release the fears you have related to abandonment, financial security, social status, motherhood, and creativity. Instead create a worry-free environment that will enable your reproductive organs to give birth to babies, books, relationships, professions, ideas, and creative works. "Whenever I see a woman with a uterine problem such as fibroid tumors, I ask her to meditate upon her relationships, creativity and sense of security," writes Christiane Northrup, M.D., *Women's Bodies, Women's Wisdom: Creating Physical and Emotional Health and Healing* (Bantam, $18.95). "Fibroids, endometriosis, diseases of the ovaries, and other pelvic disorders are manifestations of blocked energy in the pelvis."

ACUPUNCTURE

Sis, if you're anything like me, then the idea of having needles inserted into specific points of your body (that's what the "puncture" refers to in the word *acupuncture)* sounds unappealing, maybe even frightening. But acupuncture treatments are pain-free. The needles used are about the width of a strand of hair; that's superthin! So you probably won't even feel them being inserted, and if you do it won't be any worse than a mosquito bite. These days, most acupuncture needles are disposable, so you don't have to agonize over whether you're in danger of catching anything from anyone else. You also don't have to worry about side effects, unless you're dealing with a careless acupuncturist—that's why picking the right practitioner is key (see sidebar).

My first acupuncture experience was a pleasant one. I actually had a session in my hotel room when I went away on business. The practitioner arrived toting her mobile massage table and disposable needles—she was ready to work. Like a traditional physician, she had me fill out a comprehensive medical history form and talked to me to determine whether I wanted her to address any specific medical challenges. She also asked about my eating habits and other general issues. Those pleasantries are pretty typical of any acupuncture visit.

What happened next? The acupuncturist, Afua Bromley, took steps to assess my health and well-being. The diagnostic tool, the technique used to assess your overall health, depends on the practitioner's choice of acupuncture as well as training background. There are several schools— including Japanese, Chinese, Korean, and Western—of acupuncture, and each has its own way of doing things. The acupuncturist I used had studied Oriental-style techniques; practitioners of this discipline typically provide a partial physical examination during the patient's initial visit. In my case, Bromley took a quick glance at my tongue and checked my pulse (referred to as tongue and pulse diagnosis). Next it was time for the "puncture" portion of the visit. She told me to lie on the covered massage table, and I did so while remaining fully dressed—except for my shoes and pantyhose. Then she inserted the needles at different points of my body. Although there was definitely a strategy to the points (also referred to as acupoints), the selection process seemed pretty random to me. Supposedly, there are 360 acupoints where the meridians, fourteen invisible channels that serve as pathways for the life force called ch'i (pronounced "chee"), surface. Stimulating the right meridian is key because certain ones are associated with organs such as the liver and bladder. Further, the proper stimulation promotes the balance of ch'i.

Once the needles were inserted, she allowed me to relax for thirty minutes before she removed them. While I was resting she wrote up my prescription. The total time of my visit was a little more than an hour. But treatment times can vary widely and treatment visits can range from once to twice a month. In some states, acupuncturists are required to be licensed, while other states require certification by the National Commission for the Certification of Acupuncturists. In Bromley's case, her treatments are $75 for each visit, but treatment rates vary by state and whether or not the practitioner is also a physician. The good news is that a medical insurance plan may cover acupuncture treatments if they are administered by a physician.

In my case, Bromley concluded that I had fibroids. Even though I'd known this for years, I was impressed that she could spot my condition in seconds by simply eyeballing the pattern and color of my tongue—

particularly since I'd seen at least three gynecologists before fibroids even came up. Bromley believes that fibroids are the result of a poorly operating liver, which is the same theory proposed by Dr. Jewel Pookrum, a holistic gynecologist specializing in integrative medicine. She says that the liver, which is responsible for the breakdown of protein and fat, becomes stressed when it's forced to process a high-meat diet and this could prevent the proper removal of excess estrogen in the blood. The aftercare that my acupuncturist suggested included dietary changes and massaging some specific pressure points on a daily basis. Acupuncture points that relate to the uterus are found on the ankle.[1] She's convinced that using acupuncture and acupressure as well as natural teas will get results.

The good thing is that even if your fibroids don't respond to acupuncture, you shouldn't experience any side effects. Still, you should avoid this treatment if you bruise easily, have a clotting disorder, or are currently taking blood-thinning agents, because an inappropriately inserted needle could damage a blood vessel or injure nerves, organs, or tissue. If you're pregnant, avoid having the needle inserted into your abdominal area. And you should definitely avoid this treatment if you're fearful of needles.

Will acupuncture shrink your fibroids or relieve your symptoms? "The answer is maybe—though your chances are probably better if your fibroids are small," according to Johanna Skilling. It's hard to tell how effective acupuncture is for the treatment of fibroids because research suggests that women typically use this type of treatment as a last resort, "when their fibroids are too big, or their symptoms are too severe to benefit," she adds. "Some practitioners think that there are points on the body that control and prevent the growth of cells: Stimulating these points may keep fibroid cells from growing. Still acupuncture may be more consistently successful in treating pain or bleeding from fibroids [rather than the fibroids themselves]." The thing to consider is that this type of treatment isn't necessarily quick; relief could take up to six months.

The practice is promoted as a pain-relieving technique, and I've heard stories of women who say that their fibroids have shrunk. According to Chinese theory, the manipulation of the needles allows the balance and restoration of the body's life force, which is referred to as ch'i or qi. From a Western perspective, scientists claim that acupuncture releases the body's natural painkilling substances, endorphins, as well as alter the state of neurotransmitters (serotonin and norepineph-rine). Still, neither explanation has been conclusively verified.

Results aren't consistent and there aren't any concrete statistics re-garding success rates. Acupuncture can help alleviate fibroid symptoms such as pain and bloating by affecting the nervous system, which pro-motes circulation and blood pelvic congestion. But women with less se-vere symptoms are more likely to experience relief than more serious cases. There's even some dispute as to whether acupuncture provides anyone with "real" relief. An article on msn.com health (July 18, 2001) reported that by some estimates 50 to 70 percent of acupuncture pa-tients with chronic pain report some relief. But the article also states that doctors still debate whether acupuncture is any more effective than a placebo (fake treatment). This argument indicates that the ritual of acupuncture has a greater effect on patients' mental and physical state than the actual treatment. But even if that is the case, if going to an acupuncturist makes you feel better, then that should be good enough for you. On the other hand, if acupuncture is a real sticking point (no pun intended) for you, then consider the wealth of other nat-ural therapies that you can explore, including a sister-related technique called acupressure.

Moxibustion—Self-applied "Prick-less" Acupuncture for Fibroids

Moxibustion[2] was a practice used in acupuncture prior to needles. This technique requires that you burn the herb moxa (mugwort) and hold it near the various acupuncture points that affect your fibroids (see illus-tration on page 180) until the area feels hot—after a few seconds. The moxa, a fluffy woollike material that's rolled up like a thick incense, burns slowly and uses heat to penetrate areas that are unattainable by the needles. The moxa was once considered the best treatment alterna-tive for ailments and you can purchase it at a health food store or a place that promotes Chinese medicine.

Picking the Right Acupuncturist

- Get recommendations from people you trust.
- Select acupuncturists that have been certified by the National Commission for the Certification of Acupuncturists (NCCA) or the American Academy of Medical Acupuncture (for physicians).
- Request the use of disposable stainless steel needles.
- Choose an acupuncturist that has experience treating fibroids.
- Find out the other type of techniques—such as reflexology, massage, aromatherapy—the practitioner uses.
- Ask the practitioner to describe the type of follow-up you can expect before you agree to treatment.

Resources

National Commission for the Certification of Acupuncturists
PO Box 97075
Washington, DC 20090-7075
202-232-1404
202-462-6157

American Association of Acupuncture and Oriental Medicine
4101 Lake Boone Trail, Suite 201
Raleigh, NC 27607
919-787-5181

National Acupuncture and Oriental Medicine Alliance
PO Box 77511
Seattle, WA 98177-0531
206-524-3511

ACUPRESSURE

Traditionally African Americans have been resistant to consider acupressure as a viable treatment option, but the results could surprise them, according to the book *HealthQuest Staying Strong: Reclaiming the Wisdom of African American Healing* (Whole Care Health, $14). Acupressurist Yahfaw Shacor says that the reluctance her African American patients feel typically dissolves after the first treatment and they always come back for return visits. She says patients often report relief after only a few sessions. States Shacor, "I always say this: You've tried everything else; why not try a little of this?"

Like acupuncture, acupressure requires the stimulation of certain points for relief (see illustration on page 181). If used regularly, experts say acupressure can have some impact on preventing illnesses, healing, pain relief, and relaxation. The major difference here is that acupressure is needle-free. At the same time, acupressure isn't as effective as acupuncture is at accessing the points on the body.[3] But if you are particularly fearful of needles or just want to consider another natural therapy, acupressure may be a viable alternative for you.

And you don't have to rely on a professional for treatment. Although you can contact the Acupressure Institute (510-845-1059) for referrals and general information, acupressure is a technique that you can perform on yourself. In *Nature's Cures: From Acupressure & Aromatherapy to Walking & Yoga, the Ultimate Guide to the Best Scientifically Proven, Drug-Free Healing Methods* (Bantam, $6.99), Dr. George Milowe, based in Saratoga Springs, New York, says, "[Acupressure] is easy to learn, convenient for self-care and, for many, it provides real benefits." To learn techniques, speak directly to an acupressurist, read a book such as *Acupressure's Potent Points* by Michael Reed Gach (Bantam, $17.95), and try some experimenting on your own by finding points that provide you with relief.

When performing acupressure on your own or with the help of a friend, hands should be clean and nails should be clipped. Once you find the right point, probe the area using your fingertip or the second joint on your index finger. For one to three minutes, add pressure making tiny circles into the skin, then stop for a few seconds and begin again. You'll want to work on each area for five to twenty minutes at least once a day or whenever you have symptoms. During the treatment, the acupoints may feel tender, sore, or uncomfortable; this indicates that the meridian or energy pathway may be blocked. The tenderness should slowly dissolve as the treatment continues and you may feel energy begin to radiate from that area. Even if you don't, your real objective is to experience a reduction in your symptoms.

But will it help your fibroids? Dr. Susan Lark admits that "acupressure may not be as effective in women with more severe and advanced cases; these women may need to use Western medical treatments along with a variety of self help therapies." Even in less severe cases, relief may be temporary. But that may be just the remedy you need.

REIKI HEALING

Ready for more talk of energy channeling? Reiki healing, a technique that enables a practitioner to channel energy into a client for self-healing and relaxation, treats patients through a series of orchestrated touch patterns. "This is not a massage technique but more of a 'laying of hands,'" asserts an expert featured on ReikiOne (*www.reikione.com*). A full treatment lasts about an hour and the results are unpredictable, according to the web site, "the amount of energy transferred depends on the client's willingness to use it." But as with any natural remedy the results, if any, vary widely.

During my session, I laid down on a standard covered massage table. Except for my shoes, I was fully clothed. The practitioner, Karima, asked that I close my eyes and began chanting positive affirmations to promote the free flow of energy. As I lay on my back, she guided her hands about one inch above my body in an attempt to open the meridians facilitating the proper funneling of ch'i. At times she laid her hands on certain areas. The process can stimulate warm sensations throughout the body or sensations in one or more areas. For me, the one-hour session was relaxing. The results, however, remain to be seen. Adds Karima, "Fibroids can grow back even if they are taken out. Western medicine is saying that they're not sure why they develop. But Reiki healers are saying that if we address the problem in the second chakra we can get to the core and they won't grow again and give you problems. We believe that fibroids are a manifestation of something that hasn't been dealt with and when we start to deal with [the blocked energy] there is a release."

You may or may not experience any change at all. The key to any treatment's effectiveness will be determined when you assess whether your symptoms have diminished or your fibroids have reduced in size.

REFLEXOLOGY

Reflexology is a technique that you can perform on yourself at any time in any location. For this treatment method, you use your fingers to apply pressure to the correct points on your ears, hands, and feet (see illustrations on pages 182–83). According to Chinese medicine, this process will enable you to target the performance of various organs because the hands and feet, integral parts of reflexology, serve as maps to the rest of the body.

Like acupuncture and acupressure, reflexology aims to balance and restore the flow of energy because the imbalance of energy causes areas in the body to malfunction. The process is simple and harmless.[4] And unlike acupuncture, reflexology doesn't require the use of a specialist or practitioner. In some instances, doctors may even prescribe reflexology over other nontraditional treatments.

Plus, reflexology feels great, particularly on the skin. Still, its greatest value is beneath the skin, where the pressing and rolling activates a healing that travels throughout the body to renew tissues and restore cells. The warmth from the pressure triggers the release of endorphins, the neurochemicals that alleviate pain. Once done correctly, reflexology can relax the nerves, relieve discomfort, and promote internal balance.

POLARITY THERAPY

You've heard that opposites attract; that's essentially the premise of polarity therapy (also referred to as polarity balances). This technique proposes that you can experience physical, emotional, and spiritual fulfillment when your opposite energies (yin and yang) are in balance. Like Reiki healing, polarity uses the human touch (see illustration on page 184), the manipulation of energy flow, and the balancing of the chakras (see "Seven Major Chakras" illustration) to treat conditions. This technique also integrates various forms of bodywork such as yoga, self-awareness, and diet to facilitate the release of blocked energy. The practice combines Western understandings of electromagnetic power fields with Chinese, Ayurvedic, and ancient Egyptian healing practices. Under polarity therapy, the body is divided into four vertical and three horizontal zones with each having a positive, negative, or neutral charge. These zones correspond to the major chakras cited in traditional Indian yoga or the five elements (earth, water, fire, air, and ether) of Ayurvedic medicine.

A polarity therapy session will usually last between sixty and ninety minutes. It can be performed on a one-on-one basis or with a group of practitioners. Initially the practitioner will discuss your medical history, check your reflexes, and touch certain body parts (excluding your private parts, of course) to determine energy blocks. You'll then be asked to remove your jewelry (particularly metals) and shoes and lie on a massage table, the floor, or a bed. Depending on your needs, the practitioner can choose from three levels of touch in polarity therapy: no touch, where the hands are moved about through energy fields while remaining above your body; light touch; and a deep massage touch. When touch is involved, the therapist will balance the energy currents by putting his "positive" hands on a "negative" area of your body. The practitioner may also rock your body, hold your head, or massage certain points. According to the *Gale Encyclopedia of Medicine*, you'll probably need about four polarity sessions for some concrete results. This therapy will also require that you drink plenty of liquids, change your diet, and start practicing yoga.

This therapy is becoming more widely used and probably more acceptable by Western medicine because it doesn't require patients to subscribe to a specific set of beliefs or theories. It's also used in conjunction with more traditional treatments, so you can undergo polarity treatments while working with your gynecologist to treat your fibroids.

MAGNETIC THERAPY

In the *Women's Health Series: Clinically Proven Alternative Therapies for Relief from Women's Health Conditions* by the editors of *Alternative Medicine* magazine, William H. Philpott, M.D., suggests that "therapeutic-quality magnets, worn over the uterus at night while sleeping, can shrink fibroid tumor over a period of months." This occurs, according to Philpott, because the magnetic fields trigger metabolism and increase the oxygen that's available to cells, which diminishes inflammation. Although magnets may have to be applied for several months up to a year before shrinkage or elimination occurs (if at all), Philpott insists that magnetic therapy will instantly stop the tumor from further growth upon starting therapy.

For treatment, Philpott recommends that the magnets be worn over the pubic area or lower abdomen every night while you're asleep. Remember to keep the negative pole sides of the magnet facing the body because these fields are believed to normalize the body's metabolic function to treat fibroids and alleviate painful conditions. Still, using magnets is not a substitute for pain relievers or local anesthetics. In addition, you shouldn't attempt this therapy unless you first seek the guidance of a qualified practitioner. For further guidance, contact Philpott directly: William H. Philpott, M.D., PO Box 50655, Midwest City, OK 73140; 405-390-1444.

Magnet FYIs

- The magnet should be a 5"x12"multimagnet flexible mat, with a 4"x6" by 1/2" ceramic block booster magnet attached in the center of the mat with Velcro.
- Use a wrap cloth with Velcro attachments to keep the mat and booster in place on the body.
- Don't use a magnetic bed for more than eight to ten hours.
- Industrial magnets have different positive and negative poles than magnets used in medicine. Use a compass or magnetometer to determine positive and negative poles.
- Wait from sixty to ninety minutes after you eat before applying magnets to the abdomen—otherwise they could interfere with your digestion.
- Do not apply the positive pole to the body unless your doctor advises it. This can result in hallucinations, seizures, poor sleeping habits, accelerated tumor growth, and addictive behavior.

Source: *Women's Health Series: Clinically Proven Alternative Therapies for Relief from Women's Health Conditions* by the editors of *Alternative Medicine* magazine (Future Medicine Publishing, $18.95), 132.

MASSAGE

Did you think massages should be reserved for pampering purposes? Not so, according to massage therapist Genene Wellington. She believes massages should be integrated into your regular wellness program at least twice a month because the physiological effects are endless (see illustration on page 185). Internally, massages work your organs by improving blood circulation, increasing digestion, and balancing the nervous system. Massages also facilitate the healing of injuries, reduce pain, speed muscle recovery, stimulate lymphatic circulation, and promote relaxation. Externally, massages can improve posture and enhance the texture of your skin by making it smoother, softer, and more elastic. Studies by the Touch Research Institute at Florida's University of Miami also found that massage therapy can ease fatigue and chronic pain as well as other ailments.

But how can massage therapy treat fibroids? There are a couple of ways. If your fibroids are causing you to feel depressed or if you have some anxiety about an upcoming operation, get a massage to calm your nerves and help you think clearly. If your fibroids are causing aches in your back or legs, start getting regular massages to treat the pain. Generally, massages are beneficial as a companion to just about any fibroid treatment method. According to Marian Williams, R.N., in the book, *Nature's Cures: From Acupressure & Aromatherapy to Walking & Yoga, the Ultimate Guide to the Best Scientifically Proven, Drug-Free Healing Methods* (Bantam, $6.99), "Patients receiving massages require less pain medication and suffer less insomnia." So, girlfriend, you don't have to save your massage for a special occasion—book one today.

Massage Don'ts

Don't have a massage if . . .
you are pregnant, acutely ill, or feverish.
your abdomen is sensitive because you have a hernia or have eaten within the past two hours.
you have arthritic joints.
you have a rash or other skin irritations such as acne.
you have varicose veins.
you have painful blood clots in the veins (thrombophlebitis).
the area(s) you want to treat contains known tumors.
the area(s) you want to treat contains a surgical incision.

Source: *Nature's Cures: From Acupressure & Aromatherapy to Walking & Yoga, the Ultimate Guide to the Best Scientifically Proven, Drug-Free Healing Methods* (Bantam, $6.99).

To Get Your Massage On . . .

Get referrals. Collect suggestions from people you know as well as the American Massage Therapy Association (AMTA) at 820 Davis Street, Suite 100, Evanston, IL 60201; 847-864-0123; 847-864-1178 (fax).

See how it's done. Check out a video such as "Massage Your Mate" and "Massage for Health." Both VHS cassette tapes will show you how Swedish and Shiatsu techniques are performed, and you might pick up some pointers on how to sharpen your own massage skills.

Emphasize atmosphere. Your surroundings can impact the effectiveness of your massage—remember you're supposed to relax. So the location you choose should be warm, quiet (no cell phones please), and calming with soothing music in the background.

Lie on a massage table or the floor—not a bed. Despite your inclination, beds are actually a terrible place to perform or receive massages because they absorb too much pressure.

Insist on massage oil. It's a must. Vegetable oil will do, but scented oils add to the relaxation.

Speak up. Let the provider know if the strokes are uncomfortable or painful. At the same time, if the masseuse has hit the spot, communicate that too.

What can techniques of touch do?

- Improve blood circulation by alleviating muscle tension.
- Improve psychological and physical well-being by alleviating muscle tension.
- Manipulate lymphatic fluid, which promotes the release of toxins, wastes, and pathogens from the body.
- Create balance between the body's structure and function by aiding in better circulation, more flexibility, easier and more varied movements, and release of tension.
- Enhance the operation of all internal organs through improving circulation and easing tension.
- Enhance mood by improving the operation of the soma (body) which also impacts the psyche (mind).
- Reduce stress by promoting relaxation.
- Manipulate the flow of energy to promote healing.

Source: William Collinge, M.P.H., Ph.D., *The American Holistic Health Association Complete Guide to Alternative Medicine* (Warner, 1987, $24.95).

Write down your impressions about techniques of touch.

_____

_____

_____

_____

Do any of the techniques discussed in this chapter sound appealing to you? If yes, which ones and why?

_____

_____

_____

_____

Which ones are you going to try?

_____

_____

_____

_____

Date of appointment(s):

_____

Time:

_____

Name of practitioner:

_____

Location:

_____

Phone number:

_____

What were your impressions of your first visit?

_____

Would you recommend this practitioner to another sister? Why or why not?

_____

_____

_____

_____

_____

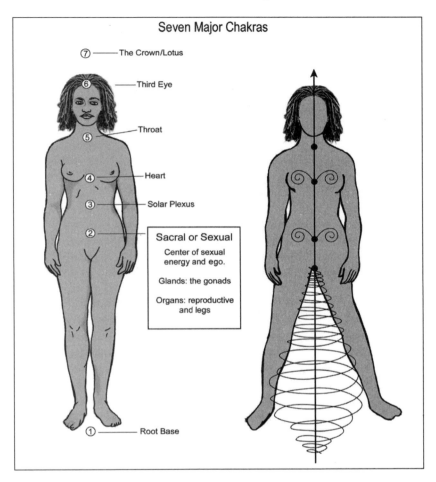

Seven Major Chakras

⑦ —— The Crown/Lotus

⑥ —— Third Eye

⑤ —— Throat

④ —— Heart

③ —— Solar Plexus

② ———

Sacral or Sexual

Center of sexual energy and ego.

Glands: the gonads

Organs: reproductive and legs

① ——— Root Base

Drawing Force

According to Christiane Northrup, M.D. in her book, *Women's Bodies, Women's Wisdom: Creating Physical and Emotional Healing* (Bantam, $18.95), the female energy is synonymous with centripetal or "drawing in" force. The earth's energy is drawn up through the feet and then spirals around the womb, breasts and tonsils as shown in the figure on the right. Therefore, you can overcome fibroids as well as other challenges because you get your power straight from Mother Earth.

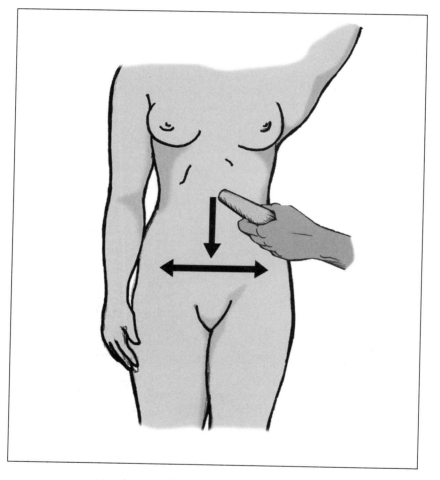

Moxibustion for "Prick-less" Acupuncture

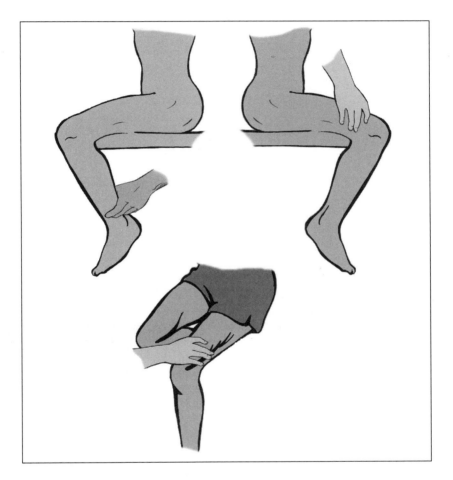

Acupressure Points for Fibroid Relief

Hand Reflexology Chart (Back of Hands)

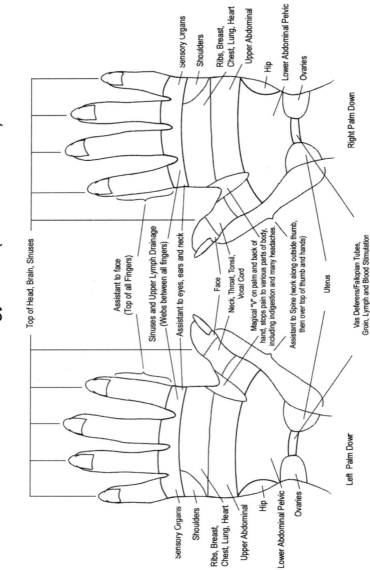

Top of Head, Brain, Sinuses

Assistant to face
(Top of all Fingers)

Sinuses and Upper Lymph Drainage
(Webs between all fingers)

Assistant to eyes, ears and neck

Face

Neck, Throat, Tonsil,
Vocal Cord

Magical "V" on palm and back of
hand, stops pain to various parts of body,
including indigestion and many headaches.

Assistant to Spine (work along outside thumb,
then over top of thumb and hands)

Uterus

Vas Deferens/Fallopian Tubes,
Groin, Lymph and Blood Stimulation

Sensory Organs

Shoulders

Ribs, Breast,
Chest, Lung, Heart

Upper Abdominal

Hip

Lower Abdominal Pelvic

Ovaries

Right Palm Down

Left Palm Down

Sensory Organs

Shoulders

Ribs, Breast,
Chest, Lung, Heart

Upper Abdominal

Hip

Lower Abdominal Pelvic

Ovaries

Foot Reflexology Chart (Bottom of Feet)

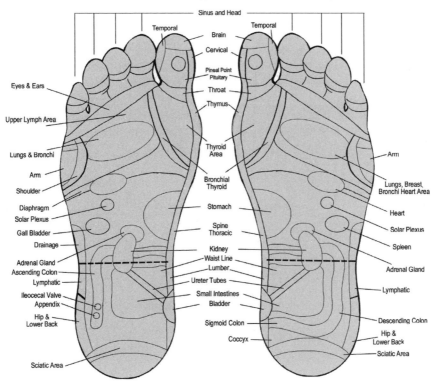

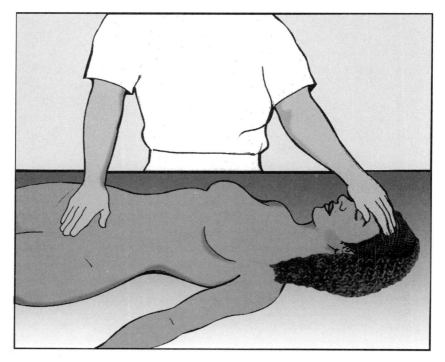

Polarity Therapy for Relief

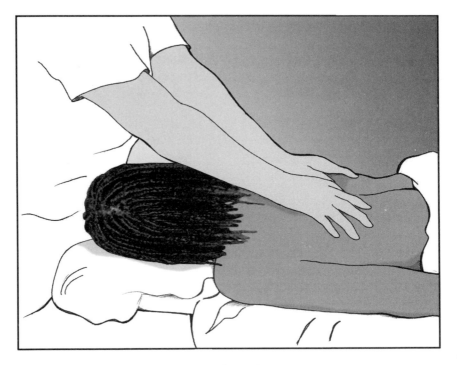

A Massage for Relaxation

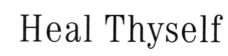

10 Heal Thyself

Prayer (and Positive Thinking) Changes Things

Someone else's prognosis doesn't have to be yours, even if you're suffering from the same symptoms. The key is in your belief system and your ability to maintain a positive attitude regardless of the circumstances that surround you. Start managing your thoughts by listening to self-healing tapes and soothing music. Also, surround yourself with people who make you feel good about yourself. Keep believing that positive thinking will reap positive results.

By the same token, understand that negative thinking can bear disaster. If you're carrying negativity around, then you better believe it's going to manifest itself in some physical way. For many black women this pessimism turns up as uterine fibroids—tumors that house anxiety, fear, resentment, self-doubt, and other stresses.

So what's a sister to do? Go back to the basics. Get down on your knees, tell the Lord about it, and leave it there. Let go and let God.

—Debbie Slater, OB/GYN Nurse Practitioner

I've never been ashamed of the gospel of Jesus Christ, and I've been taught to believe that anything is possible through faith and prayer. That's why I asked for supreme guidance from the very instant I found out about my fibroids. As a result, I feel that my choices as they related to the treatment of my condition were ordered by the Almighty. Still, I'd be lying if I didn't admit that I was afraid, nervous, and upset every step of the way even with prayer in the midst. On the other hand, prayer made the unbearable a little more bearable and gave me hope when I could have wallowed in despair. I am a living witness: prayer changes things.

But if you need proof, there are a host of studies that promote the power of faith and prayer. One article found that individuals who are part of organized religions have a greater tolerance for stress, tend to live longer, and seem to have a lower rate of sickness and disease and this appears to be due to their faith in a higher being. A 1998 study by the San Francisco General Medical Center found that coronary patients who were prayed for were five times less likely to require antibiotics and three times less likely to develop cardiopulmonary arrest than the coronary patients who weren't prayed for. In addition, Pastor A. R. Bernard, spiritual leader of the Christian Cultural Center, a ten thousand-member church based in Brooklyn, New York, cites several women who say they have cured their fibroids as well as other feminine problems through prayer. "There is medical evidence where doctors report that a disease existed, a growth existed, a malady existed and after prayer it was gone and they could not explain it," he says. "Years ago, my own wife had a cyst on her ovary the size of a grapefruit. After we had prayed about it in the church, the same doctor who diagnosed the cyst found that it was gone when he went in to deliver my son through cesarean section. There was no explanation. We have other accounts in the church and we can provide documentation."

Further research by medical institutions is underway. Medical schools such as Harvard, Johns Hopkins, and Georgetown are dedicating a portion of their curriculum to the study of religion and medicine. The historically black Morehouse School of Medicine in Atlanta now offers spirituality courses to its medical students. Plus, other researchers throughout the United States have established institutes to further study the correlation between prayer and healing.

But we black folks have always known that "God (Jehovah, Lord, Father, or whatever term you use) is a doctor that never lost a patient" and we've called on his assistance from the beginning of time. Repeatedly we've listened to testimonies touting miraculous recoveries from breast cancer, high blood pressure, alcoholism, and diabetes. That's what we've heard, but do our actions show that we actually believe those stories? Or do we doubt that those miracles are for us?

If so, then it's time that our behavior line up with what we truly believe. One thing is for sure: incorporating prayer into your treatment regimen for your fibroids has its benefits even if your tumors don't go away. According to Bernard, "Prayer takes you to a higher level where you are not bound by the realm of humanity's weaknesses and limitations. Calling on the divine, God, immediately gives you a sense of hope and not futility because you are now appealing to someone who is not bound by time, space, sickness, or disease and that has an immediate impact on your thinking."

So how can you make positive thinking and prayer work for you and your fibroids? Here are some suggestions:

EXAMINE YOUR BELIEF SYSTEM

What are your beliefs about healing? If you're a woman that has grown up around family members who have constantly been ill, you may have come to believe (if only on a subconscious level) that being sick or having fibroids is normal. During my saga when I visited several physicians I was told repeatedly that almost "every black woman you know has fibroids" as if it was a normal state. Even though that statement was supposed to be some form of consolation, it made me furious. For one thing, it made me feel that the issue of fibroids wasn't a concern among the medical community particularly since they have yet to discover a cause or cure for them. As far as I was concerned, their prevalence only showed that there needed to be more research done to treat fibroids—a condition that I considered to be a serious problem and in no way "normal."

But that was my take on the matter. Maybe you've been told that fibroids run in your family and you feel that your condition is inevitable. That's not the case. Genetic predisposition is not an inevitable "sentence"[1] that dictates that you will get a particular disease or condition. According to Christiane Northrup, there are numerous cases where women do have a strong family history of fibroids and have been healed of the conditions or never even developed them. That's because there are environmental factors that largely influence whether a predisposition is ever expressed. Further, your attitude affects your health condition as well as the approach you take when challenges develop. Sis, you have more power over your fibroids than you think. But first you have to believe that you deserve to be fibroid-free.

BE HONEST ABOUT THE PURPOSE YOUR FIBROIDS
ARE SERVING

Sounds crazy? I bet you're wondering what purpose your fibroids could possibly be serving if all you're getting is grief. Well, have you ever considered that grief is what you want? Being in pain, out of touch, cranky, or downright miserable prevents you from being accessible to participate in other things—maybe activities that you'd rather do without anyway. Instead of taking a "mental health day" from work, you were able to take off because you were having trouble with your fibroids. Or rather than tell your sweetie that you weren't in the mood for lovemaking, you could blame it on your troubling fibroids. Don't be ashamed. As Northrup points out in her book, society looks at meditation, napping, or cooling out as being irresponsible. In addition, some of us only get the attention we crave from our loved ones when we are ill. As a result, we begin to feel that the only time it's socially acceptable for us to rest and be nurtured is when we're sick. Adds Northrup, "Being sick in this culture can be a very powerful way to get our needs met legitimately. Saying to someone, 'Please hold me—I feel ill' is quite different from saying 'Please hold me—I want to be held because it feels good and I like it.' The first sentence uses illness to justify the universal human need for closeness. The second sentence simply states the need clearly."

It took me some time to admit that some of the best times I'd had to myself were during the times I was in the hospital being treated for my fibroids. Are you kidding? Dinner was prepared and I didn't even have to worry about the dishes. Fresh flowers, which I absolutely love, arrived like clockwork. My visitors were genuinely concerned about me—not about what I could do for them—and were in a good mood. Plus, the few phone calls that I received were pleasant and not related to work. Except for a few aches and pains, life was good.

And there is nothing wrong with my appreciating the things that I value such as feeling loved, receiving flowers, and getting phone calls from friends that express general concern. There was something wrong, however, with not being honest about what I needed and relying on my fibroids to get me the results. Honesty required that I let people know that I'd appreciate it if they didn't call me at home for work-related issues unless it was an emergency. I also revel in reaching out to friends for a hug from time to time. What do you need? Start being honest about these things and get the love you deserve.

FORGIVE AND FORGET

Sounds like a cliché? Perhaps, but learning to forgive and putting the past behind you is essential to true healing. Fibroids, some say, are nothing more than balled-up resentment and anger, so holding on to negative energy can destroy your uterus. Now, forgiveness doesn't mean that you condone someone's behavior. It simply means that you've released the hurt associated with those actions so that it can no longer adversely affect your life. Forgiveness frees us to experience the joy that awaits us.

How do you forgive? There are several ways, but you can develop your own ritual for forgiveness. For example, find a quiet secluded place where you can meditate on that person and tell them verbally or through a letter that you forgive them. Then give up all feelings of resentment toward them. Vow never to concentrate on what they did to you again. Most importantly, stop shaping your behavior toward others in response to that previous experience. Stop saying or insinuating things like "all men are the same" and treat people as individuals. In addition, sincerely wish the person that offended you the best that life has to offer, even if you think they don't deserve it. Now, forgiving someone doesn't mean you give them a green light to further abuse you, so don't continue to repeat the same unhealthy behaviors of the past that resulted in your disappointment. At the same time, show your trust that God knows best by letting go of the anger, hatred, resentment, jealousy, and fear—forgive.

STICK WITH THE FACTS

This has been a personal challenge for me. Typically when I hear news, I immediately categorize it as being good or bad. Some things just "are what they are." But at times we pass judgment on a scenario and view our conclusions as facts. That's a bad habit to have because our response isn't based on accurate information.

If your gynecologist has confirmed that you have fibroids, then that is a fact. If your follow-up tests have provided information about the size and location of your fibroids, then those details are also facts. However, since there are no definitive explanations about what actually causes fibroids, everything else is mere speculation. You cannot conclude that your fibroids are a punishment from God, are a result of your having a previous abortion, are indications of your evil spirit, are signs that you shouldn't be sexually active, or are a reflection of any other personal shortcomings. Now, that's not to say that you shouldn't take whatever steps you feel are necessary for relief, but trying to determine what part of your behavior is to blame for these tumors is pointless. Focus your energies on remedying the situation, not wallowing in it.

THINK POSITIVELY

I know this is easier said than done, but what other choice do you have? The only way you can truly gain control of your behavior is by remaining positive. Otherwise, you'll get caught in a web of emotions that could be detrimental to your health. Alternatively, a positive attitude can strengthen your immune system and facilitate a speedy recovery. Further, you get back what you give in life. When you smile, you'll notice that people smile back at you. At the same time, when you try to maintain a positive attitude you'll receive positive reactions from others—including the people that you need for support like your physician, family, and friends. Writes Johanna Skilling, "Creating a positive attitude in the people around you can reflect right back to you, like a smile in the mirror."

And you never know how your reaction can change someone's life. I'll never forget a story I saw on the news many years ago. A Trinidadian woman visiting New York was robbed on a subway train and thrown on the tracks. Although the woman lived, both of her legs were severed and she was never going to walk again. Now, that woman would have had every right to be furious, upset, angry, and hateful. She was minding her own business when a young thug targeted her for madness. Yet she gave a positive response when a news reporter asked, "Are you sour on New York because of your terrible ordeal?"

"Of course not," she said. "This is just something that happened.

New York is still a wonderful city with plenty of opportunity. I'm not only glad to be here in New York, I'm glad to be alive because things could have been much worse. Thank God for his blessings."

My life was forever changed by that moment. If that lady could smile and speak positively after having both of her legs severed while being on vacation, then what the hell was I complaining about?

VISUALIZE GOOD HEALTH

In the book *Women's Bodies, Women's Wisdom: Creating Physical and Emotional Healing* (Bantam, 1998, $18.95), Dr. Christiane Northrup suggests that you picture yourself at optimal health as a first step toward healing. By imagining a fibroid-free uterus, you force your mind to develop a plan to live up to your expectations. "If we can change the consciousness that creates our cells, then our cells and lives improve automatically, because health and joy are our natural state," insists Northrup. A. R. Bernard agrees and says prayer and visualization provide our bodies with a frame of reference, "so our mind, spirit and body come in line with what we pray for. That's a part of the healing process."

According to Susan M. Lark, M.D., in her book *Fibroid Tumors & Endometriosis: Solving Problems of Heavy Bleeding, Cramps, Pain, Infertility, and Other Symptoms* (Celestial Arts, $16.95), visualization exercises serve as a mental blueprint for a healthier body. To remedy fibroids, Lark suggests you use the "erasure" imagery to help you visualize the melting away or disappearing of your tumors.

COMBINE PRAYER WITH ACTION

Faith without works is dead, according to James 2:20. Healing takes "prayer and action," insists Dr. Barbara L. King, a metaphysical author and minister at Hillside Chapel and Truth Center in Atlanta, Georgia, who was featured in the book *Staying Strong: Reclaiming the Wisdom of African American Healing* (Whole Care Health, $14). Although she says prayer was responsible for the successful removal of a lump in her throat, she admits that following a strict herbal and nutritional program prior to the surgery was also helpful and warns that prayer by itself is not enough. "You have to follow through with an act of faith," she says.

That could mean changing your diet, getting regular checkups, joining a gym, and starting other activities for better health.

And don't pray for answers if you're going to ignore the response you get. Sometimes the higher power provides us with all of the information we need to better our lives, but we don't like the advice. True healing may require that we exit an unfulfilling relationship, ditch a dead-end job, or enlist new friends. Change is scary but not impossible. So step out on faith and believe that the divine guidance you receive will lead to a better tomorrow.

SELECT A DOCTOR WHO SUPPORTS YOUR BELIEFS ABOUT HEALING

"If the doctor is a believer, then it strengthens your prayer because you become united," states Bernard. So your ability to maintain a positive attitude isn't the only factor that's critical to the healing of your fibroids. Your physician's beliefs also play a role in the outcome of your therapy. According to Larry Dossey, M.D., author of *Healing Words: The Power of Prayer and the Practice of Medicine* (Harper, $6.50), the best scenario for healing is when you and your physician genuinely believe that a treatment is going to result in a positive outcome. At the same time, if there is conflict between the two sets of beliefs, then that presents the worst situation. According to Bernard, "If the doctor is exercising faith and the patient praying is exercising faith then that prayer becomes empowered even more so."

That's why Dossey strongly suggests that you find out about a doctor's beliefs before becoming his patient. You don't need to subject your doctor to an interrogation or a long list of questions to determine his beliefs, cautions Dossey. Simply answer the question, "Does the doctor make me feel better or worse when I'm around him or her?"

And don't forget that finding the right doctor is also a supreme gift. Your healing doesn't have to come in the supernatural. Perhaps God is using the doctor as a healing tool. "Sometimes there may be a misunderstanding about medicine and religion on the patient's part," says Morehouse School of Medicine's Dr. Clay. "They may believe it's a lack of faith to be treated by a doctor, but if you talk with them and help them understand that God gives doctors knowledge to help people heal, you can clear up any misunderstandings."[2]

That said, I also suggest that you openly discuss your beliefs about prayer and ask whether the physician minds if you incorporate it as part of your treatment. For example, the two of you can have prayer before an examination or treatment therapy or after a discussion. If your physician is strongly against prayer, then maybe that's not the physician for you.

DON'T UNDERESTIMATE THE POWER OF YOUR UNCONSCIOUS MIND

"We will never be able to take full advantage of the power of the mind to shape our health—including the mind's use of prayer—until we broaden our concept of 'consciousness,'" writes Dossey. That means we must acknowledge that there are forces operating on our behalf that may be beyond our capacity to fully understand—it's a commitment to believe in the things we cannot see or hear. In doing this, we give our unconscious mind permission to help us achieve good health. Adds Dossey, "The unconscious mind can initiate or cooperate with prayer and even mediate the effects."

One active means of controlling the unconscious mind is through hypnosis. In her book, Johanna Skilling suggests that hypnotherapy can be used to treat the pain and discomfort associated with fibroids, to minimize pain before surgery, and as a relaxation method. One practitioner offered hypnosis as a means for controlling excessive bleeding and pain, proposing that women can achieve relief by visualizing their blood vessels stopping the blood flow. If you're considering this treatment, you can see a qualified hypnotist (see resource listing) or hypnotize yourself by setting some time aside to talk to yourself (literally) and establishing a new reality for your fibroid condition.

Other ways to get in touch with your unconscious mind include keeping a journal (discussed below), meditating, and saying affirmations. I recorded a few affirmations on a tape recorder that I play back every morning. This helps me start my day off on a positive note because I start to internalize some of the phrases. What types of things would you like to accomplish each day? Write them down and say them out loud. Also get in the habit of reciting positive talk (see "Affirmations" sidebar) so you can start your day off on the right foot. Just be sure your affirmations aren't all talk, cautions Bernard. "Affirmations are powerful but affirmation without discipline leads to delusion," he insists. "I can affirm something but if I don't discipline myself and bring my actions, words, thoughts, and motives in line with those affirmations, then I'm deluding myself." So make sure your affirmations are supported by action.

Start tapping into your unconscious mind by meditating over a list of questions, which include:

- At what age did you discover you had fibroids?
- What circumstances were prevalent in your life at that time?
- What people were present in your life at that time?
- What was your emotional state just before you were diagnosed with fibroids?
- Were you in the center of any trauma or stress at that time?
- How were those issues resolved? (If they weren't resolved, then develop a strategy to change the circumstances or accept they are beyond your control.)

KEEP A JOURNAL

What's on your mind? Whatever it is, write it down. Recording your thoughts, feelings, and insights will help you build a stronger connection with your brain, higher power, and uterus. It also allows you to determine how your emotional state impacts your physical condition. In addition, the process may help you discover what your fibroids are trying to tell you or what you need to release so that your fibroids will go away. Says Bernard, "Disease is not only a matter of what you eat but what's eating you." Keeping a journal can help you uncover what's eating you so those issues can be resolved and purged out of your system.

According to Debrena Jackson Gandy, in a *Black Enterprise* article ("Don't Worry, Be Happy," July 2001), you should set aside at least ten minutes a day to write in your journal and be willing to devote more time if other opportunities develop. Keep a flashlight, tape recorder, pen, and pad by your bed in case you wake up with some ideas or thoughts during the night. Also, if a word or phrase continues to pop up in your head, don't ignore it. Write it down, meditate on it, and wait for the universe to reveal its true meaning to you. In addition, get in the habit of recording any details that you can remember about specific dreams. All of these actions confirm your commitment to getting to know yourself and healing.

READ THE SIGNS

"To rely on a single approach, no matter how philosophically or metaphysically attractive it might be, is to court disaster," says Larry Dossey. He says that believing in the power of prayer isn't a green light to deny the obvious. Since no approach is 100 percent effective, it's important that we pay attention to the signs and insights of others as well as our own. If we continue to try an approach that continues to be ineffective, then that could indicate that it's time to try something else. Also, healing through prayer may not come in the form that we expect, so you shouldn't close your mind to a remedy that you may have initially opposed. Adds Dossey, prayer, like other healing techniques, must be "used wisely."

Reading the signs means we maintain a connection with our physical and emotional state. Biologically, we are programmed to respond to environmental stimuli in tangible, physical, and measurable ways.[3] For example, in times of fear, our bodies will either "fight" or "flight." Our muscles tense up and breathing becomes short and quick. So if the divine guidance you think you received causes intense physical reactions, then maybe you've misunderstood the message.

GET HELP

Sometimes true healing requires a team effort. Aside from talking to your physician, you may want to bend the ear of a close girlfriend or boyfriend (yes, they might even be helpful). They could have access to information that you need or could direct you to another resource.

And don't underestimate guidance from a therapist, a psychiatrist, or even a stranger. People who know you the least can provide objective feedback and introduce you to new life strategies and techniques. Besides, they may be the tool that the universe has decided to use to help you make your health decisions.

RECRUIT OTHERS TO PRAY FOR YOU

"The more people that you can join in faith, the more powerful your prayer becomes," advises Bernard. I second that statement and am a firm believer in starting a prayer chain for the restoration of mental or physical health. When I'm going through things, I'm not ashamed to ask someone to send some prayers up on my behalf, and I also pray generously for others. As the Bible says (Matthew 7:7): *Where two or three are gathered in my name they can ask anything and be granted.*

Submit your fibroid concerns, for prayer to your church. I know it's not as serious as some of the other concerns, but you're entitled to healing too. Get support from the women in your Bible study group. Or get a prayer partner. The two of you can commit to reading the Bible and praying once a week.

So how can prayer and positive thinking help you heal your fibroids? The possibilities are endless. All you have to do is believe in those possibilities and make a commitment to make them happen.

What affirmations do you want to make about your fibroids? Here are some examples. Then feel free to develop some of your own. Recite all of them at least once a day and repeat the ones that are most important to you at least three times. Don't forget to record them on a tape cassette so you can play them on a regular basis.

AFFIRMATIONS FOR FIBROID HEALING

- I have a healthy uterus.
- I am fibroid-free.
- I am pain-free.
- I have a normal menstrual cycle every month.
- My uterus is a normal size and shape.
- My estrogen level is normal.
- My menstrual cycle is one of God's glorious blessings.
- I enjoy a well-balanced healthy diet.
- I enjoy a healthy exercise program.
- I am stress-free.
- I am at peace.
- I love my body.

- I am ready for the fruit (whether it's a baby, novel, idea) that my uterus is destined to produce.
- My body, mind, and spirit are in balance.
- My life coincides with God's purpose for me.

Write some other affirmations that apply specifically to your needs:

_____

_____

_____

_____

_____

_____

11

Pillow Talk

How Fibroids Can Affect Your Sex Life

Girl, I've been married for sixteen years and I enjoy looking good for my husband. I have always been shapely, had a small waistline, and liked being sexy for him. But my fibroids made me look about four months pregnant and I felt that I had lost my sex appeal. I just lost all interest in sex until my husband told me that I was still very sexy and he desired me now more than ever.

Still, I just could not continue life this way. I wanted my LIFE BACK!! I met with an OB/GYN who discussed my options in detail. I decided to have the uterine artery embolization (UAE) or uterine fibroid embolization (UFE). After the procedure, I noticed an immediate difference. My doctor, John Lipman, informed me that my cycle would go back to normal after a few months. It has not gone back to normal completely, but I suppose that's a gradual process. I can feel my cycle getting a little lighter month by month, my stomach getting flatter week by week, and my energy level increasing day by day. In the words of James Brown, I feel good!!!

—Leslie E. Royal, Age 35, Freelance Writer and Publicist

Sis, there isn't anything sexy about pelvic pain, vaginal bleeding, or feeling an excessive desire to urinate while you're trying to enjoy intimacy with your partner. Although fibroids and the symptoms that accompany them may not have any impact on your sex life, they have been known to put a damper on the evening's festivities if you're one of the unlucky ladies that are affected by them. Says Johanna Skilling, "If your fibroids are too large, sex can be painful, or just, well, weird."

There are various ways that your fibroids could cause some unwelcome interruptions. For one thing, fibroids can make you feel less feminine if your abdomen has become enlarged. Also, the crowding that fibroids can cause in the pelvic area can make it difficult for the uterus to properly contract during an orgasm, causing pain and discomfort. In addition, fibroids can cause pain, bloating, pressure, and other discomforts that may make sex less pleasurable. And if fibroids are affecting your fertility or preventing you from using certain forms of contraception due to the distortion of your uterus, this could also cause you to opt out of a sexual encounter. Further, if you're worried about whether having intercourse will cause vaginal bleeding, that fear alone may cause you to hold off on sex, and if you fail to express your concerns you may leave your partner feeling rejected, sparking a host of other difficulties in the relationship. And if your fibroids tend to bump up against organs like the rectum or bladder during intercourse, that sensation could throw things off kilter. Although these shifts won't cause you any physical harm, the activity could cause discomfort for you and your partner—just ask him!

In any case, don't let your fibroids wedge an emotional and physical barrier between you and your partner. You have a right to good sex and so does your partner. Instead of letting fibroids overcome you, view your myomas as an opportunity to discover how your body works, an incentive to find the sexiest treatment options available, and a challenge to create more ways of enjoyment for you and your partner.

SEXUAL RESPONSES IN YOU

"Good sex is a whole body experience," writes Johanna Skilling. Touching and allowing yourself to be touched is a way to trigger physical responses in yourself and your mate as well as build an emotional bond between the two of you. Orgasms can spring up in different areas of your body, including the clitoris, vagina, nipples, skin, or brain. "Even paralyzed women, who have no feeling below the rib cage, are capable of having an orgasm," Skilling adds. So if you don't want your fibroids to keep you from getting the best orgasmic response ever, you need to know how your body works to get that response. Take a lesson:

Your Blood

Alrighty now, once you've been sparked, the adrenaline starts flowing and your blood starts rushing to different areas such as the uterus, vagina, and pelvic muscles. The swelling of blood is behind the tingling sensation that you feel when you get wound up.

The Uterus

Once you're sexually stimulated, your uterus starts to pull up and backward toward your spine and lengthens the vagina about an inch. It also swells up to twice its normal size. When you have an orgasm, you may feel your uterus contracting as the muscles clench and unclench, causing the pressure inside of the uterus to increase. And according to experts, a great orgasm is associated with the pressure change in the uterus.[1]

A uterine orgasm seems to be heightened when "your G-spot, a coin-sized nerve center in the front wall of your vagina, is stimulated," according to Skilling. Your uterus may also respond when your nipples are pinched, sucked, or fondled. What you need to know is that the uterus is a key component for multiple orgasms. When the initial swelling from your first orgasm stays in place, this keeps you geared up for round two, three, and so forth.

The Cervix

Don't discount the use of opening the uterus as a source of sexual pleasure. The cervix, a donut-shaped disc located at the entrance to the womb, releases beta-endorphins during intercourse, chemicals that can block pain, heighten your arousal, and increase your pleasure.

The cervix also produces half of the lubrication that you feel when you're having sex—the vaginal walls produce the other half. There's also a theory that the vagus nerve, a nerve that shoots from the cervix to the brain stem, is a pathway for orgasmic sensations.

The Ovaries

Ovaries release androgens, hormones that increase sexual arousal. Your ovaries also maintain the proper lubrication in your vagina and keep your vaginal walls strong.

The Brain

Have you ever let an orgasm pass you by because you were preoccupied? We all have and that's proof that no amount of physical stimulation can get you aroused if your mind is somewhere else.

FIBROID TREATMENTS AND YOUR SEX LIFE

So you've decided to get treatment for your fibroids and you're wondering just how this treatment will affect your sex life? Generally speaking, if your fibroids have been causing some interference things should get better. As one doctor told me, "If you've been bleeding and in pain on most occasions, you probably aren't having much sex anyway." Still, you should talk to your gynecologist to discuss any concerns that you have about how your treatment will affect your sex life before you go under the knife or start taking any drugs. Your physician, however, can give you only a general indication as to what symptoms you can expect. Each patient is different, and you may not know the full range of symptoms until you actually undergo treatment. Still, here's what other women have experienced after these treatments:

Drug-Based Therapies

Gonadotropin-releasing hormone (GnRH) agonists, commonly consisting of either Lupron (leuprolide acetate) or Synarel (a brand name for GnRH agonist nafarelin acetate), stunt fibroid growth and even shrink them by cutting off the production of estrogen. The problem with these treatments is that your body is thrown into menopause and you suffer all the symptoms associated with it. So get ready for the side effects that come with reduced estrogen such as hot flashes, weight gain and bloating, moodiness, loss of bone density, vaginal dryness, and a reduced sex drive. The good news is that doctors use drugs to treat fibroids only for short periods (three to six months) because of these intense, at times dangerous, side effects. Once you stop the treatment, however, your body along with your sex drive should go back to normal.

Uterine Artery Embolization (UAE)

There is limited information that suggests that sexual pleasure is actually improved for UAE patients. An article on streetdoctor (*www.streetdoctor.net/women-can-have-better-sex.htm*) reported findings from a study presented at the Society of Cardiovascular and Interventional Radiology in San Antonio, Texas, which stated that "43% of the [UAE patients] reported an increase in sexual desire after the procedure." The trouble with this statement is that the study was based on only twenty-one UAE patients. In addition, it's unclear whether the improved sexual response is due to relief from the uncomfortable symptoms that are associated with fibroids or an improvement in the woman's orgasmic response. "Even with this small sample of 21 patients, the findings were statistically significant," says Dr. Michael G. Wysoki. The current study also found that 43 percent of gynecologists changed their thinking about embolization to either favorable or indifferent after their patient underwent the procedure and that younger female gynecologists are more receptive to UAE. This may be an indication that this procedure could become more popular in years to come. Fortunately, Wysoki indicated more research on this topic using a greater number of participants.

Since UAE operates by slowing the flow of blood to the uterus, it can affect women with uterine orgasms—roughly one-third of all women.[2] A segment of these women say their orgasms aren't the same following UAE. One reason a woman could have problems with orgasms following UAE is if the nerves going to the uterus have been damaged. "If you embolize and block the blood supply to the nerves going into the uterus, those nerves may very well be damaged," states Dr. Scott Goodwin in Skilling's book. And if you were feeling something in your uterus that was pleasurable, you may no longer feel that after embolization."

But again, not every woman experiences uterine orgasms, so this may not apply to you. Plus, each case is unique and much more research needs to be done in this area for some definitive results.

Myomectomy

I must admit that I was a little gun-shy after this procedure, and I've heard that from other women as well. Doctor's orders are that you should refrain from sexual activity for at least six weeks, but I was trying to run the "no-sex" marathon because I was afraid that my uterus couldn't sustain the sudden impact. Boy, was I wrong. To my pleasure, I found that things were never better. My uterus could contract without the fibroids causing foul play such as pain, pressure, or bleeding—these symptoms were a thing of the past. And my tummy was flatter than ever and that made me feel sexy again. Other myomectomy patients also report dramatic improvements after the procedure.

Hysterectomy

According to Herbert A. Goldfarb, author of *The No-Hysterectomy Option: Your Body—Your Choice* (Wiley, $15.95), 40 percent of women indicate a reduced sexual response after a hysterectomy. First of all, the decreased estrogen causes physical changes in the sexual organs, including a shortened, less expandable, drier vagina—this alone can make intercourse painful or uncomfortable. The vagina may also alter because of the development of scar tissue or because it is shorter and tighter. In addition, the absence of the uterus assures that the contractions associated with intense uterine orgasms are a thing of the past. What's more, the removal of the cervix means that lubrication is largely diminished and the physical sensation derived from the beta-endorphins it produces is also eliminated. Both of these factors could make intercourse particularly painful. Further, the removal of the ovaries promotes more reduction of lubrication as well as diminished testosterone and androgens, hormones that play the most significant roles in arousing your sex drive. And although a study of nearly seven hundred women found that those that kept their ovaries had a much better attitude toward having a hysterectomy than those who didn't, it appears that your ovaries need the uterus for survival. About a third of the women with a hysterectomy experience an ovarian shutdown. Finally, one study showed that a hysterectomy affected all types of sexual behavior including hugging, kissing, touching, and even daydreaming.[3]

Now there are artificial hormones and lubricating jellies to deal with the physical sexual changes that may accompany a hysterectomy. K-Y Jelly, for example, is a water-based lubricant that may facilitate moisture for pain-free intercourse as well as stimulate the body's own lubricating mechanisms. Estrogen restores lubrication and the tone in the vagina. Progesterone treatments can decrease depression and testosterone can pump up the sex drive, although its intake should be monitored due to its negative side effects. Just don't expect these aids to do as good a job as your own body has done all of these years. "Lubricating jellies restore wetness to the vagina, but they do nothing to replace the lack of arousal that would have stimulated the vagina to become lubricated in the first place," notes author Susanne Morgan in Goldfarb's book *The No-Hysterectomy Option: Your Body—Your Choice* (Wiley, $15.95). So you certainly shouldn't go into any surgery, particularly a hysterectomy, with the idea that you will feel the same as you did in the past. Adds Goldfarb, "you may feel the same; you may feel better; or you may feel worse."

Beyond the physical challenges, women with hysterectomies may have to deal with the emotional and psychological difficulties that they or their partners have to face. For some women, the womb is symbolic of their femininity, youthfulness, and liveliness. The loss of the uterus as well as the loss of menstruation can be disturbing and may even cause them to feel less attractive and incomplete. Other women, however, are able to enjoy a smooth transition. To ensure the best outcome for you, make sure that you are confident that a hysterectomy is the right choice. And be honest about your feelings regarding this procedure. "A caring partner, friend or even therapist can help sort out your fears and feelings," advises Skilling. Organizations such as Hysterectomy Educational Resources and Services (HERS; 610-667-7757) located in Bala Cynwyd, Pennsylvania, can provide you with support through their twenty-four-hour counseling sessions, newsletter, and various other resources. Or consult a nurse at your doctor's office or at the hospital where you plan to have your surgery to talk about your concerns about sex after surgery. "Consider this part of your life just as carefully as you would any other aspect," adds Skilling. "Make sure your doctor understands and shares your concern—and interest—in you having a happy, fulfilling sex life."

Of course you can't enjoy sex to the fullest unless you consider the feelings of your mate as well as your own. Just as you have fears and concerns about how a hysterectomy may influence your sex life, the man in your life may also have them. Confront your partner about his concerns before having the hysterectomy. And if the two of you decide to move forward with the procedure, discuss these concerns again. Men may be affected by the physical and emotional changes that happen to you. In addition, the reduced lubrication and diminished elasticity may make intercourse more difficult and less pleasurable for him. "Instead of dismissing or ignoring any negative feelings, come to terms with them," advises Goldfarb.

PEAK PERFORMANCE

So how can you ensure you have great sex no matter which treatment option you choose? Keep in mind that great sex starts in the brain, not the bedroom. Take some time out to think about some creative ways to enjoy a sexual encounter with your mate—even if you choose not to have intercourse due to troubling fibroids. Carlita Figueroa-Faxton, author of *Getting Him, Keeping Him, Making It Work* (C. Figueroa, $7.50), offers these suggestions for heating things up in the bedroom:

- **Compliment your mate when you're alone or with others.** Regardless of the company, speak highly of your mate. Spread the word about how wonderful he is and he'll live up to your expectations.
- **Make love to his senses.** Romance him with your favorite song in the background, recite poetry to him, burn incense, or whisper sweet things in his ear. This builds anticipation and stimulation.
- **Look the part.** "Don't wear rollers, scarves or turbans to bed. Your hair should be clean, free of anything sticky, greasy or oily; your body should be clean, soft and smooth, free of superfluous hair," insists Figueroa-Faxton. She also says you should ditch the flannel pajamas and slumber only in a silk, satin, or lacy tricot number that's wrinkle-free and lightly scented. Adds Figueroa-Faxton, "Seduction is a mental process which began with the physical attraction you both felt when you first met. That image and aura should be enhanced."
- **Intoxicate him with your fragrance.** Choose a scent that you both like and watch out for the sparks. He'll be on a mission to sniff you out—literally. You can also relish in knowing that he'll think about you whenever that aroma hits his nostrils, whether you're in his midst or not.
- **Maintain good manners and a pleasant disposition.** Leave the attitude at home, girlfriend. Smile, soften your eyes, and listen attentively to what your man has to say. Men find charm quite appealing and a pleasant attitude makes for the start of an enchanting evening (or morning, for that matter).
- **Dance daringly.** It doesn't have to be Sadie Hawkins night to ask your man to dance. Simply put on some soft music, put your arms around him, and do your thing. With your looks, charm and sweet smelling fragrance, how can he resist?
- **Build anticipation.** Leave a sexy note where you know he'll find it. Place a napkin drenched with your favorite perfume in his

briefcase. Send a coded e-mail that only the two of you under-stand. All of these things let him know you're game for romance. Says Figueroa-Faxton, "The 'chase,' and the 'wait' and the antici-pation are part of seduction."

- **Inject the unexpected.** Massage and fondle his thumb. Suck his finger. Nibble on his ear. Make out in unusual places as if you were naughty teenagers. Attack the vein popping in his neck as if you were a vampire. This type of excitement will keep the fire flaming.

- **Become a master of a great massage.** Rub your mate's mid-section, rub his feet, or run your fingers through *his* hair. Ac-cording to Figueroa-Faxton, "your hands should be in constant motion all over his body: kneading, squeezing, massaging, fondling, gently pinching, smacking and spanking. Make him feel as though you have suddenly grown tentacles like an octopus."

- **Be on the lookout for new ideas.** Get as much information as you can to help you heat the sheets. For starters, read *The Joy of Sex* and *How to Make Love to the Same Person for the Rest of Your Life*. Also sneak a peak at the adult sections of your neigh-borhood book and video stores, you might see something inter-esting and pick up pointers.

- **Keep a positive attitude.** If you're suffering from fibroids, they can definitely get the best of you—if you let them. That's why it's important that you stay upbeat so you can prevent your condition from ruining the intimacy between you and your partner. If inter-course is uncomfortable or painful, try some of the strategies here for some sexual stimulation and excitement. Also, don't wait for problems to start before you start making your sex life a prior-ity—start today.

List ten positive things you can do for your mate. Next to each, write a date when you plan to take action. Then, just do it!

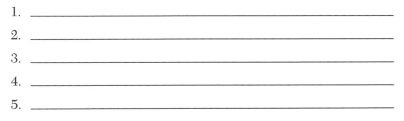

1. _____

2. _____

3. _____

4. _____

5. _____

6. _____

7. _____

8. _____

9. _____

10. _____

List ten positive things you can say about your mate, then get in the habit of communicating these items to him as well as others:

1. _____

2. _____

3. _____

4. _____

5. _____

6. _____

7. _____

8. _____

9. _____

10. _____

12 Copycat Syndromes

Other Conditions Resembling Fibroids

It's a good thing that I had a myomectomy. When I looked at the report from the operation, it indicated that the surgeon came across endometriosis. That's another condition that can cause heavy bleeding, infertility, and abdominal pain. She said she tried to remove as much of it as she could.

Gee, if it weren't for the surgery I wouldn't have even known I had that condition. I probably would have blamed all of my problems on fibroids.

—Peaches

So far we've discussed the symptoms associated with fibroids, traditional as well as nontraditional methods for treating them, and how these menacing myomas can impact your fertility and sex life. By now, you probably think you know enough about fibroids to diagnose yourself. Right? Wrong. "Any condition that produces a mass effect in the pelvis may cause the same type of pressure system as fibroids," remarks Richard W. Henderson, M.D., F.A.C.O.G., an OB/GYN based in Wilmington, Delaware. There are also a host of conditions that cause the same type of symptoms as fibroids such as heavy painful bleeding, painful intercourse, lower abdominal pain, urinary tract infection, and bowel blockage. So it's best to let your doctor make the diagnosis, says Henderson. "An examination will give you an idea of what type of abdominal mass you have," he adds. "Your doctor could also perform a CAT scan or MRI but an ultrasound is the best choice."

Even if you do have fibroids, that's not to say that your symptoms can't be caused by another condition as well. After I had my surgery, one of the attending physicians told me that he'd removed a polyp, a fingerlike overgrowth of cells, from my uterus. Like fibroids, this condition can cause abnormal bleeding. Without insight from a gynecologist I wouldn't have had a clue that I'd even had this condition. This information is significant because the treatment options for polyps could be very different from treatment options for fibroids.

To arm you with valuable insight, this chapter offers descriptions, symptoms, and treatment options for a selection of conditions that may mimic fibroids. The information highlighted here is not meant to scare you but to provide you with the tools to inspire your physician to consider other alternatives. Let's take a look at how conditions such as ovarian cysts, ovarian cancer, ectopic pregnancies, uterine cancer, polyps, endometriosis, and adenomyosis could impact your health.

OVARIAN CYSTS

"An ovarian cyst is simply a collection of fluid within the normally solid ovary," according to William H. Parker, M.D., author of *A Gynecologist's Second Opinion: The Questions and Answers You Need to Take Charge of Your Health* (Plume, $13.95). They are extremely common among women, but it's important to remember that ovarian cysts rarely require treatment because they typically go away on their own and are rarely cancerous. Ovarian cysts may or may not cause discomfort, and as with fibroids, most women discover that they have them during a routine examination.

Many cysts don't cause any symptoms. However, there are those that cause pelvic pain or pressure as well as abnormal periods if the cysts interfere with the production of the hormones (estrogen and progesterone) that regulate your menstrual cycle. Abnormal menstrual cycles could consist of periods that are either too heavy or too light and that are too long or too short. Irregular hormone levels caused by cysts can result in breast swelling or tenderness, water retention, and intensified PMS-type symptoms. The good thing is that once the cyst dissolves or is removed, your period and your body should return back to normal within one or two cycles.

Infertility is associated with cysts in two ways. One culprit is the endometrioma, an ovarian cyst that contains endometriosis cells. This type of cyst causes blood to settle within the ovary and can prevent a woman from getting pregnant. Although it's unclear how this type of cyst specifically causes infertility, there are theories attempting to offer some explanation. It's believed that endometriosis cells generate chemicals that prevent the ovary from releasing an egg or interfere with the sperm's ability to fertilize the egg. Also, severe endometriosis may cause scar tissue that hinders the egg from passing through the fallopian tubes.

Another cyst-related condition associated with infertility is polycystic ovary disease (PCO), also referred to as Stein-Leventhal syndrome. Under this condition, multiple small cysts develop in response to hormonal changes. The numerous cysts (which are about a quarter of an inch in size) can enlarge the ovaries by two to three times their normal size. Your erratic periods might be a sign of PCO. Other symptoms include hair growth on the face, high blood pressure, deepened voice, enlarged clitoris or ovaries, obesity, oily skin, acne, and infertility. As a first line of defense, the drug clomiphene is used to treat infertility that's associated with PCO.[1] But if conception doesn't occur after the first three months of using clomiphene, your physician should try other treatments.

Just how are ovarian cysts diagnosed? Your doctor should come across them during your pelvic examination. Typically the ovaries are the size of a small walnut. However, when cysts are present, the ovary is enlarged and the growth is a movable, soft lump. Physicians can't differentiate among the four types of cysts during an examination, and at times "it can be hard to distinguish between an ovarian cyst or tumor and a myoma. A gynecologist doing a pelvic exam asks herself: Is it a myoma, an ovary, a cyst or a tumor?" writes Yvonne S. Thornton, M.D., M.P.H., in her book *Woman to Woman: A Leading Gynecologist Tells You All You Need to Know About Your Body and Your Health* (Plume, $13.95). One way to make a determination is by manipulating the uterus, she states. If the growth moves with the uterus, "[it] is most likely a myoma. If not, it can be a pedunculated myoma—a myoma attached to the uterus by a stalk—or it can be an ovarian tumor."

If you haven't gone through menopause and the cyst isn't bothering you, you can use the wait-and-see approach. The key here is to see how the cyst behaves during a follow-up visit. If the cyst dissolves after two or three weeks, then no other treatment is necessary. If the cyst remains intact, however, the doctor should schedule a test such as a sonogram to determine a treatment plan. "The most accurate way to get a picture of the ovary and cyst is with a vaginal sonogram," advises Parker. "Depending on which cells in the ovary are overgrowing, certain types of ovarian cysts will make fairly reliable patterns on a sonogram."

Your treatment options depend on the diagnosis. Surgery may be required if your cysts are causing you severe pain, indicate cancer on a sonogram, or fail to decrease in size after eight weeks. The strategy here is to remove the cysts before they continue to cause more discomfort or grow to the point of destroying the ovary. Certain types of cysts such as follicular, corpus luteum, and hemorrhagic typically go away by themselves, while endometriomas, epithelial (serous, mucinous), and dermoid cysts are noncancerous masses that require surgical removal to prevent damage to the ovary. Further, cancerous cysts which may come in the form of epithelial or germ cell cancers need to be surgically removed, and patients may have to undergo other treatments as well.

OVARIAN CANCER

Ovarian cancer is rare. Only one out of every fifteen thousand women age thirty and under will have this disease. One out of every ten thousand women will have this disease by age forty. And one out of every fifteen hundred women will have ovarian cancer by age sixty. If you have not gone through menopause and your doctor finds a cyst, it's probably benign. There's even a 70 percent chance that an ovarian cyst is benign in a woman that has already entered menopause. So if a growth is found or your ovaries have become enlarged, don't panic.

Even so, it's important that you receive annual gynecological exams so that any changes in the size of the ovary can be detected. Aside from some minor complaints such as bloating, pelvic cramps, or abdominal irritation (which may come from a number of intestinal issues), there are no early warning signs for ovarian cancer. The majority of ovarian cancer sufferers (60 to 70 percent) have already reached the advanced phase of the disease by the time they are diagnosed.

ECTOPIC PREGNANCIES

In ectopic pregnancies, the fertilized egg starts to develop in the fallopian tube rather than the uterus. Conditions such as scar tissue or endometriosis may block the passage of the egg to the uterus. This condition is dangerous. Unlike the uterus, the fallopian tube does not have the ability to accommodate a growing fetus. So once the embryo starts to grow to about the size of your thumb in diameter, the fallopian tube will begin to tear, causing abdominal pain.

Fortunately an ectopic pregnancy can be diagnosed before the fallopian tube is damaged. If the pregnancy hormone human chorionic gonadotropin (HCG) does not continue to increase as expected, an ectopic pregnancy or miscarriage is suspected. Your doctor may also be able to detect an ectopic pregnancy upon examination because the fallopian tubes may have a tender swelling. In any case, examination, HCG blood testing, and sonogram ensure that this type of complication is found much earlier than it has been in the past.

Laparoscopic surgery enables the physician to remove the pregnancy tissue to prevent it from further damaging the fallopian tube. There is also a drug called methotrexate used to destroy the placental tissue in early ectopic pregnancies.

UTERINE CANCER

Uterine cancer is the most common type of cancer in the female pelvis. Still, the condition is very rare. It's almost nonexistent in women under age thirty, with sixty being the average age of uterine cancer sufferers.[2] Women who are nulliparous (have never had children), overweight, diabetic, hypertension sufferers, or taking estrogen without balancing it with progesterone are the diseases's major victims.

The condition develops when the cells of the uterine lining (or endometrial cells) begin to grow in an abnormal, uncontrolled manner. For this reason, uterine cancer is often referred to as endometrial cancer, and the terms *endometrial cancer* and *uterine cancer* have become interchangeable. There are two stages of uterine cancer: the precancerous phase (or atypical endometrial hyperplasia) and the cancerous phase. Fortunately, each of these stages can be successfully treated if they are diagnosed early. The abnormal overgrowth of precancerous or cancerous cells can be detected under a microscope. The cells appear abundant, crowded, and irregularly shaped. In addition, the portion of the cell containing the genetic material starts to divide faster than usual.[3] But these abnormalities can't be detected unless a woman sees her physician. Since the early stages of uterine cancer are not accompanied by nausea, pain, vomiting, or other symptoms, it's important that any abnormal vaginal bleeding be considered as the first sign for further testing.

Keep in mind, however, that most women who experience irregular bleeding do not have uterine cancer. But since the cells of uterine cancer sufferers become particularly fragile, they tend to bleed. So you should see your physician immediately if you experience irregular bleeding at any stage of your development—whether you just started having periods, have been having them for years, or haven't had them in quite a while. Postmenopausal women have the highest incidence of uterine precancer or cancer, so any irregular bleeding should send them straight to their gynecologist's office. "The shedding may occur month after month or it may happen only once," advises Thornton. "If it is just once and the woman is not sufficiently attuned to the significance of irregular bleeding to consult her doctor, then she may miss the single warning of the presence of uterine cancer."

Treatment for precancerous uterine cells may depend on whether or not you desire to have children. If you do want to have children and want to avoid a hysterectomy, you can try to take high doses of progesterone. Sometimes this hormone can eliminate the condition before it worsens. Progesterone is given as a pill for a period of three months; then a D&C is performed so that the remaining cells can be tested. As a follow-up, repeated endometrial biopsies and D&Cs are performed to ensure the cancerous cells don't return. Your physician may also prescribe a treatment for the hormonal imbalance that caused the growth of your precancerous cells in the first place.

If progesterone treatments do not cure your condition, if you aren't considering having children, or if your condition has already progressed to the cancerous stage, a hysterectomy is strongly recommended. In fact, "a hysterectomy cures 95 percent of women when the cancer is found early," notes William H. Parker in his book, *A Gynecologist's Second Opinion: The Questions and Answers You Need to Take Charge of Your Health* (Plume, $13.95). In some instances, radiation may also be used to treat this condition.

POLYPS

It is unknown what actually causes these grapelike overgrowths of cells that may be found in the intestines, nasal passages, and uterus.

However, the important thing to know about polyps is that they are very easy to diagnose in your gynecologist's office and are rarely cancerous when found in the uterus.

Your gynecologist can see exactly where these growths are located by inserting a very small telescope called a hysteroscope into your womb. Typically, polyps are loosely attached to the uterine lining and can be easily removed by D&C or with a small grasping instrument in your doctor's office under local anesthesia. Upon removal, the hysteroscope is reinserted to ensure that the growths have been completely removed. In some instances, hospitalization and anesthesia may be required if the polyps are large or they are attached to the lining of the uterus by thick stalks. In this case, a resectoscope may be used to remove them. Polyps typically grow slowly and even though they can grow again after they are removed, regrowth usually doesn't occur until years later.

As with fibroids, small polyps may not cause any symptoms. However, as they begin to grow they could cause bleeding and fertility problems. Since polyps can be malignant, although rare, your physician may do a Pap smear to ensure that the growths are benign. Major surgery is rarely required as a treatment option for polyps unless they are found to be cancerous.

ENDOMETRIOSIS

Endometriosis, a condition in which cells that line the uterus start to grow in the wrong places, is the number-one gynecologic condition in the United States. It's estimated that five million women have this illness and experts say it appears to be becoming more prevalent. Between 1965 and 1984, approximately two million women had hysterectomies for pelvic pain that was caused by endometriosis. During that time, the number of hystectomies that were performed doubled each year. Annually, endometriosis is behind a significant number of women that require hospitalization. Further, endometriosis has been implicated as the primary cause in 30 percent of infertile women.

In endometriosis, misplaced tissue is primarily found in areas outside the uterus such as the ovaries, fallopian tubes, vagina, the outer surface of the womb, and other places in the abdominal cavity. At times, endometriosis may be spotted on the bladder or bowel. Or in rare instances, the condition can show up in sites as far away as the lungs.

The trouble with these misplaced cells is that they respond to the same hormones (estrogen and progesterone) as the cells in the uterus. They build up as if they are preparing for a fertilized egg and bleed at the end of the cycle when the level of estrogen and progesterone drops. But since these cells are in the wrong place, there's no place for the blood to go, so it builds up inside the body. This accumulation can cause irritation, pain, or injury to the surrounding areas. The body's response is to form scar tissue around the offending tissues, but this just causes more discomfort and may cause blockage in places such as the fallopian tubes and the ovaries contributing to fertility problems.

Treatment for endometriosis may be drug-based, surgical, or a combination of both. Oral contraceptives (a combination of progesterone and estrogen), for example, may provide relief if taken continuously because they prevent bleeding and manage the body's hormones as if the uterus were already housing a fertilized egg (pseudopregnancy). Taking the pill alone reduces the amount of blood that is shed and that can prevent the backup that may cause excess blood to be released through the fallopian tubes. Lupron, a synthetic form of the gonadotropin-releasing hormone, prevents the pituitary gland's production of FSH and LH. As when taken for fibroids, this drug throws the body into a menopause-like state where you'd experience hot flashes, vaginal dryness, mood swings, depression, headaches, and loss of bone density. After medical therapy, there is a 50 percent recurrence rate.[4]

As far as surgical remedies are concerned, the adhesions and implants from endometriosis may be removed by laparoscopy or laser beam. After a laparoscopy, there is a 40 percent chance that the endometriosis will return.[5] Larger or more widespread endometriosis may require treatment by abdominal surgery (laparotomy). All of these above procedures are considered conservative. A hysterectomy, however, is a more radical approach where the removal of the ovaries and uterus can provide the greatest relief with little chance of recurrence.

ADENOMYOSIS

Adenomyosis, a noncancerous condition related to endometriosis, occurs when the endometrial tissue within the uterine lining begins to grow within the muscular wall. Typically there is a barrier between the deeper layers of the uterine wall and the endometrium that prevents this condition. However, women with adenomyosis don't have this defense mechanism. Like the cells in the uterine lining, the misplaced cells bleed during menstruation and this may cause pain or discomfort. In addition, the buildup of blood results in inflammation of the surrounding muscle that transforms into fibrous tissue (adenomyoma) in reaction to the irritation.

Adenomyosis is often confused with fibroids because sufferers of both conditions may experience similar symptoms such as cramping, pelvic pain, an enlarged uterus, and heavy bleeding. Plus, adenomyomas look very similar to fibroids on sonograms. An MRI may be a better tool for accurately diagnosing adenomyosis, but the test is rarely used because it's so expensive. According to William H. Parker, author of *A Gynecologist's Second Opinion: The Questions and Answers You Need to Take Charge of Your Health* (Plume, $12.95), "surgery is the only way to establish the diagnosis of adenomyosis with certainty. Once removed, the tissue can be examined under a microscope."

The good news is that the condition is far less common than fibroids, occurring in about 10 percent of women, and 40 percent of women with adenomyosis have no symptoms. On the flip side, when adenomyosis is present it's typically in conjunction with other reproductive problems such as fibroids, so diagnosis may take some detective work by your physician. Unlike fibroids or endometriosis, adenomyosis seems to be more associated with women who have given birth at a late age, typically in their forties and fifties. Other theories say genetics play a role or blame the condition on a hormonal imbalance. "The bottom line is that no one knows exactly what causes it," states M. Sara Rosenthal in the book *The Gynecological Sourcebook* (NTC/Contemporary, 1999).

Initially, adenomyosis is treated the same way as endometriosis—patients are prescribed oral contraceptives, danazol, painkillers, and progesterone and told to sit tight until menopause. Adenomyosis may also be treated with the drugs Lupron and Synarel for relief from excessive bleeding and cramping. In addition, these drugs may shrink the swelling within the uterus. The problem is that, just as when these drugs are used to treat fibroids, the solution is temporary. Once the drug is discontinued, the symptoms return. Surgery is the only long-term treatment for this condition. If the adenomyosis is confined to isolated parts of the uterine muscle wall, then those areas can be surgically removed. Otherwise, a hysterectomy is recommended.

13 Oh Baby!

How Fibroids Can Affect Your Fertility

In 1995, my doctor told me that I had a small mass of fibroids. They never caused me any problems so we did not do anything about them. In 1997, I became pregnant. When I was twelve weeks, my friend took me to the emergency room because I was having severe pain and cramping. I thought that I was losing the baby. The emergency room physician really did not know what was going on. I explained to him that I had fibroids and he said that "maybe" that was the reason for my discomfort.

A few days later, my doctor did an ultrasound and said that [the fibroids] were getting larger and were causing the cramps. She said that she would not prescribe any medication during the first trimester because that is when the baby was developing his brain, heart, and other major organs of the nervous system. She did not want to take any risks and neither did I. So I was bedridden and missed many days at work because of the excruciating pain. When I reached the fifth month, all I felt was a little pressure and the pain eased up. I guess maybe the baby pushed the fibroids in different directions. On January 30, 1998, my son Bryson Denard was born. Right after his birth, I had a few months of very heavy bleeding. But since then, [the fibroids] shrunk. In fact, a recent ultrasound shows that they are smaller and I haven't had any more problems or pain. Now, I'm not considering having any surgery because the fibroids aren't bothering me.

—Lisa Kirk, Age 36
Student at Georgia State University and Substitute Teacher

S is, experts say that fibroids generally do not prevent pregnancy. In a published study, fibroids were cited as the sole cause of infertility in only 9 percent of patients.[1] In *Uterine Fibroids: What Every Woman Needs to Know* (Physicians and Scientists Publishing, 1996), author Nelson H. Stringer states that "infertility caused by fibroids is rare." On the other hand, there is a high rate of spontaneous abortion and infertility among women who have fibroids.[2] So what does that mean to you? It's hard to tell unless you've already started trying to conceive.

Just be aware that fibroids can wreak havoc at every stage of your pregnancy from preconception to delivery. Large fibroids are the biggest culprits, "treatment is usually recommended when the tumor is larger (about the size of a 12- to 14-week pregnancy), as it is likely to cause some complication eventually," note Dennis Brown, M.D., and Pamela A. Toussaint in their book *Mama's Little Baby: The Black Woman's Guide to Pregnancy, Childbirth and Baby's First Year* (Plume, $16.95). But smaller myomas, depending on their location, can also cause problems.

Still, every woman is different. And your situation can change as your fibroids continue to grow. So no one—not even your physician—can make any solid predictions about how your fibroids will affect your pregnancy. They can only make their best guess. Just know that fibroids, particularly if they are large, can interfere with the implantation of the fertilized egg, distort the uterine lining or fallopian tubes, alter the position of the cervix or ovaries, or prevent sperm from properly maneuvering in the uterus. Still, there are numerous women who conceive without difficulty and go on to have successful pregnancies. Again, you won't know which category you fit into until you test your fertility—and this should only be done when you are mentally, physically, and financially ready to have a child.

That said, this chapter will look at how fibroids can impact your ability to conceive as well as your pregnancy. It will also include suggestions for how you and your physician can deal with these challenges.

THE CONCEPTION COUNTDOWN

My gynecologist says it's time for me to face my fibroid issues—not because of a biological clock—but because of a biological truth. The fact of the matter is that you can't biologically have a baby if you have a hysterectomy and she doesn't want me to wait until the removal of my uterus is my only option. According to her, the fibroids in my uterus are taking up too much space and there would be very little room for a new addition if I became pregnant. As it stands, I would run the risk of having a miscarriage or premature labor if I conceived.

So if I want motherhood to be in my future—and I clearly do—then I need to act sooner rather than later.

But I don't know what to do. On the one hand, I could choose to have the fibroids surgically removed so that I protect myself from having a hysterectomy later but at the same time, this surgery does run the risk of resulting in an emergency hysterectomy should I run into complications. The only thing I'm sure about is that this whole scenario is driving me crazy. No matter what I pick, there's still no guarantee I'll have the baby that I've always wanted.

—Dee Dee, Age 35

Maybe you've already started trying to conceive, and when that time of the month rolls around you're wondering whether you should go to the drugstore to pick up a box of . . . well, you know. But like clockwork, Aunt Flo arrives because once again you're not pregnant so you'll actually put those feminine products to use—again. Could your fibroids be the cause of your conception delay?

Possibly. Infertility is defined as the inability to conceive after one year of unprotected, well-timed intercourse or the inability to carry a successful pregnancy.[3] If you're a woman of reproductive age, you should probably consult a fertility specialist after six months of attempting to conceive. According to Stringer, the location of your fibroid has a lot to do with just how much havoc it can cause when you're trying to become pregnant. Intracavitary fibroids (myomas that are projecting into the cavity of your uterus), for example, can cause infertility by altering the surface of the endometrial cavity, which prevents the zygote from attaching or causes the sperm to have to travel a longer distance to reach the egg. This type of fibroid as well as numerous fibroids pushing their way into the uterine cavity may block the blood supply to the fertilized egg once it's already attached, causing it to abort.[4] Fertility issues may also be the result of intramural fibroids that cause blockage of the fallopian tubes and prevent the egg from reaching the uterus. In addition, fibroids located on the top portion of the uterus (corpus) are known to cause higher incidences of spontaneous abortions than myomas located in the lower portion of the uterus.[5] There are also some experts that claim the possibility of miscarriage is very high when a fibroid is directly under the uterine cavity and is located on the same side as the pregnancy. Alternatively, the incidence of miscarriage is reduced when the fibroid is on the opposite side of the pregnancy but the woman might experience significant—sometimes debilitating—pain.

The size of your fibroid(s) is another important factor. During pregnancy, fibroids can grow by as much as 32 percent due to increased levels of estrogen. Smaller fibroids typically don't cause much trouble during pregnancy. Large fibroids, however, can be especially challenging for the patient and the doctor because they can cause miscarriage(s), premature birth, or hemorrhaging after delivery. But again, you won't know that your fibroids are causing infertility problems unless you've tried to become pregnant *and* there isn't another more likely explanation for the infertility. There may be other culprits behind your inability to become pregnant, such as endometriosis (which accounts for a significant proportion of infertility cases),[6] salpingitis (infection or inflammation of the fallopian tubes), adhesions that could be blocking your fallopian tubes, or a host of other issues that may even include your partner's low sperm count—so have him tested too!

Top Strategies Your Fibroids Could Be Using to Prevent You from Becoming Pregnant

Stop and block: If you have one or more fibroids blocking, compressing, or interfering with your fallopian tubes, this could make it impossible for an egg to make its way to your uterus. The result could be infertility or, in rare instances, an ectopic pregnancy, a critical situation where the egg begins to develop in the fallopian tubes.

Transform landscape: Fibroids can make for a bumpy landing for a soft zygote, and this hard, cold uninviting surface can prevent it from properly attaching itself to the lining of the uterus (endometrium).

Launch chemical warfare: Sort of. Fibroids can trigger the release of prostaglandin, the hormone that causes pain and the contraction of the uterine muscle—another scenario that makes it difficult for the zygote to take root.

Seek and destroy: The rapid cell division of your fibroid signals your immune system to kick in tactics to fend off the invader—your fertilized egg could get caught in the crossfire.

Source: Johanna Skilling, *Fibroids: The Complete Guide to Taking Charge of Your Physical, Emotional, and Sexual Well-Being* (New York: Marlowe & Company, 2000), 182–85.

A PAUSE FOR PREGNANCY

Hold on: if you've gotten to this stage it's apparent that your fibroids haven't caused you to be infertile. But they can still cause some problems. As we said earlier, fibroids can increase in size during pregnancy in response to the woman's increased estrogen level—although most women don't experience any change in their fibroids. According to Stringer, fibroids have receptors that receive and process estrogen. Fibroids with a large number of receptors tend to show significant growth when exposed to high estrogen levels during pregnancy. Alternatively, fibroids with few receptors are not affected by estrogen levels. Unfortunately, there is no test that can assess the number of fibroid receptors to make predictions about growth. However, we do know that large fibroids can cause miscarriage, premature labor or birth, or postpartum hemorrhage.[7] And that's not all: fibroids can cause a host of other side effects during pregnancy. The key thing to remember is that not every symptom happens to every pregnant woman with fibroids, so you may never experience any of these. But even if you do, most of them can be managed if you get immediate consultation from your physician.

Bleeding

This side effect is one of the more common symptoms for women with fibroids whether they're pregnant or not. According to the American Nurses Association, you should consult your physician for any vaginal bleeding that occurs while you are pregnant. Just be aware that a little bleeding or spotting during the first trimester can be normal.

Red Degeneration

The death of a fibroid is called red degeneration because as it outgrows its blood supply it turns a reddish or salmon-pink color. The breakdown of the fibroid can be an excruciating process that may require the woman to be hospitalized for a short period of time. This typically occurs around twenty weeks but could happen at other times during the pregnancy. The pain starts at the base of the fibroid and may spread to your lower back. You may also experience some nausea, vomiting, a low-grade fever, and light bleeding—call your physician. As

Johanna Skilling points out, the worse thing that could happen from degeneration is hemorrhaging, shock, or preterm labor, but these are not common occurrences. The good news is that relief usually follows in response to bed rest and pain medication (such as ibuprofen) after one to two weeks. But don't take any medication without first talking to your physician, and never take ibuprofen after thirty-four weeks, according to Dr. Hilda Hutcherson in her book *Having Your Baby: For the Special Needs of Black Mothers-to-Be from Conception to Newborn Care* (Ballantine, $12.95).

OVERCROWDING

"If a myoma is growing inside your uterine cavity, you can conceive but the two structures are vying for the same space," warns Yvonne S. Thornton, M.D. Crowding can increase the size of your uterus by three to five times. That means you'll get larger sooner and you'll start to experience various symptoms such as heartburn, shortness of breath, hemorrhoids, back pain, and varicose veins sooner in your pregnancy. Worse-case scenario: the cramped space could cause your fetus to suffer poor development of various body parts. But Thornton says most of these deliveries go without a hitch and "the majority of women with myomas are just fine."

PLACENTA PREVIA

In a normal environment, the placenta will develop at the top of the uterus away from the cervix. However, if your fibroids are taking up too much space in your womb, that may cause the placenta to adhere to the lower part of your uterus in between the baby and the cervix. The danger of this disorder, which happens to one in every two hundred pregnant women,[8] is that "the baby's food and oxygen source, may 'deliver' before the baby," according to Dennis Brown and Pamela A. Toussaint. Signs of this condition should be taken very seriously because you could develop severe bleeding, which could put you at risk for infection and deprive your baby of the oxygen needed for proper development. For your safety, your doctor should avoid pelvic exams to keep from worsening the condition. And you'll have to hold off on sex for the rest of your pregnancy, but just let your honey know that the sacrifice will be well worth it.

Your doctor could choose to treat placenta previa by putting you on bed rest or even by putting you in the hospital. Since there is the possibility of premature labor, your doctor could also put you on drugs to slow this process. And if things seem particularly dangerous or you've passed your thirty-seventh week, your physician may induce labor or perform an emergency cesarean. There are cases where the placenta moves again and resolves its misplacement on its own. Even in these instances, the chances are high for an early delivery.

TEAR OF THE MEMBRANE OR UTERINE RUPTURE

In rare instances, the added pressure your fibroids put on the delicate membrane surrounding your fetus causes it to rupture or break. One sign of a damaged membrane is leaking amniotic fluid. You'll feel a gush of fluid escape from your vagina that will be followed by drips. This condition puts you at risk for infection and premature delivery so call your physician right away.

Under less common, yet extremely critical, circumstances, women who have had previous surgeries on their wombs (such as a myomectomy, myolysis, or cesarean section) and numerous children (five or more) are at risk for uterine rupture during labor. Your body will warn you if your uterus is in danger of rupturing. "If you are in labor, your contractions will usually stop, you may feel faint, and you will feel a tearing sensation as well as severe abdominal pain," according to Brown and Toussaint. As a precaution, your doctor will perform an emergency C-section to secure the baby and repair your uterus. However, there are extreme instances where the uterus cannot be repaired.

SPECIAL DELIVERY

When you've gone through a dramatic life-changing fibroid experience, any live birth is extra special. If you've gotten this far, it looks like you're home free and you're probably at the homestretch of parenthood. But be aware that the presence of fibroids should compel your physician to plan for and expect the unexpected. Here are some incidences that could occur during labor and delivery in response to fibroids:

PREMATURE LABOR

Girlfriend, I hope you don't wait until your fortieth week to prepare your hospital bag, because if you're a pregnant fibroid sufferer you have a higher risk of delivering early than your fibroidless counterparts. Of pregnant women without fibroids, approximately 6 percent went into premature labor. Pregnant women with two-inch fibroids had a 20 percent occurrence of premature labor, while pregnant women with fibroids that were three inches or larger had a 28 percent incidence of premature labor.

Doctors try to treat premature labor by using drugs to slow contractions or admitting the pregnant woman in the hospital for several weeks. Premature babies can suffer from underdeveloped limbs and are even at a higher risk for death. So it's important that you contact your physician at the very first sign of premature delivery.

BREECH AND TRANSVERSE BIRTHS

The presence of fibroids may cause the baby to remain in a breech or transverse position. A baby is considered breech when it fails to rotate itself to the head-first (cephalic) position for delivery, typically by the eighth month. When breech, the baby will sit feet first or buttocks first as it did at the beginning of the pregnancy. When a baby is in a transverse position, it is lying across the birth canal. Both conditions make natural delivery extremely difficult. As a result, doctors prefer cesarean deliveries.

C-SECTION

Make no mistake, cesareans (the number-one operation among all women)[9] are more common in pregnant women with fibroids (39 percent) than in those women without fibroids (17 percent).[10] As Skilling points out, there are a host of ways fibroids can increase your chances of getting a C-section. For example, fibroids located in the lower part of your uterus may hamper the baby's descent into the birth canal. Or fibroids may keep your uterus from contracting properly, and that could prevent the normal progression of labor. Also, prior surgeries such as a myomectomy or myolysis may make your uterus too weak to sustain labor. And as stated previously, fibroids can prevent the baby from properly positioning itself for delivery.

And cesareans, no matter how common, are not without risks. You could develop an infection, experience excessive bleeding, or not respond well to a blood transfusion or anesthesia. Your baby could also have a reaction to the general anesthesia, but doctors do have ways to treat this rare occurrence. The important thing to know is that a cesarean is a serious operation that should only be chosen when absolutely necessary.

Don't assume that you are automatically a candidate for a cesarean delivery just because you have fibroids, Thornton insists. Every woman and her circumstance is unique. "I believe we should wait until she comes full term before we make the call," Thornton recommends. "Most of the time the myoma has resituated and the baby's head is bigger than the myoma so the baby floats right out." This could happen to you too.

POSTPARTUM HEMORRHAGE

Bleeding can be a problem after any delivery, but women with fibroids experience a greater incidence of this complication. Myomas may prevent the uterus from properly contracting the muscle fibers to seal off bleeding arteries so the vessels don't shut off and bleeding increases. Adds Skilling, "If you've suffered from placental abruption, premature labor, or uterine rupture as a result of your fibroids, you may also be at risk for postpartum hemorrhage."

To treat this condition, your doctor might perform a vigorous massage on your abdomen to help the muscles contract and close up the exposed blood vessels. He could also pack your uterus with gauze, inject you with a medication to slow bleeding, or seal your arteries. As in the case of a myomectomy, excessive bleeding could lead to a hysterectomy.

Doctor's Telltale Signs of Infertility

Here are the tools your physician uses to determine if fibroids are behind your infertility:

- An ultrasound (sonogram) reveals whether fibroids are altering the wall of the uterus.
- Hysterosalpingography (HSG) is used to determine whether or not the fallopian tubes are blocked. Just be aware that false-positive results can occur 20 percent of the time because a spasm can appear as a blockage. So if your doctor finds that your fallopian tubes are blocked, you may have to confirm the results with another test. The good news is that you need only one tube open for conception.
- Hysteroscopy tells whether the fibroid is affecting the lining of the uterus.

Fibroids and Pregnancy		
Stage	*Contact Your Doctor If You Have the Following Symptoms*	*Possible Results*
Before Conception	Inability to conceive for six months with well-timed intercourse	Infertility, miscarriage, ectopic pregnancy
During Pregnancy	Bright red vaginal bleeding Pain that occurs suddenly and doesn't subside Tender uterus Early contractions Excruciating pain Excessive urination Pain on the back of the thigh Tiredness	Placenta previa, a condition where the placenta adheres to the lower portion of the uterus between the cervix and the baby. Red degeneration (fibroid is outgrowing its blood supply) Pressure on bladder Sciatic pressure Anemia
After Pregnancy	Severe pain Abnormal bleeding	Fibroid is degenerating The uterus may not be contracting as it should

14

No Baby!

Contraceptive Choices for Women with Fibroids

From the time my periods started at age sixteen, I had problems. Initially, I would have it one month and miss the next two months. When I did have my period, I had severe cramps but I never knew what caused them.

Years later when I went to the doctor for my six-week checkup after giving birth to my daughter, he told me that I had fibroids. I didn't have a clue what my doctor was talking about, but he explained that it was a small growth that could be causing my bad cramps and heavy bleeding. He then prescribed birth control pills as a way to regulate my period and help my symptoms. It worked. My fibroids didn't grow and the problems with the heavy bleeding and cramping stopped. My physician told me that if the fibroids didn't bother me I shouldn't bother them so I left them alone. I think the birth control pills kept my fibroids in check.

—Margaret Brown, Age 59, Retiree

Sis, I know that we all have different views about children and motherhood. Maybe you already have all the children you could ever want, or afford for that matter. And even if you are like me (wanting to hear the pitter-patter of little feet more than anything), you'll be in the market for birth control at some point. And then there are those of us that just can't imagine starting a family—not even in the long term! The bottom line is that each of us has to evaluate birth control at some point in our lives.

I share your dilemma. Fortunately "there are a full spectrum of contraceptives," explains Richard W. Henderson, M.D., F.A.C.O.G., an obstetrician/gynecologist based in Wilmington, Delaware. In the United States the top five most common forms of contraceptives are sterilization, the pill, condoms, the diaphragm, and natural family planning, according to the Alan Guttmacher Institute, a nonprofit organization that focuses on sexual and reproductive health research policy analysis and public education in New York and Washington, D.C. "The reversible ones are birth control pills, which is by far the number one choice and Depo Provera (a contraceptive injection) weighs in at number two. Older women may use permanent sterilization. The number one non-reversible contraceptive is tubal ligation. Condoms are way down the list as a primary method of birth control, maybe third or fourth overall. . . . It's a matter of individual choice."[1]

So what are your contraceptive choices as a fibroid sufferer? "All forms of birth control—from the pill, which has side effects and has been linked to serious illnesses such as breast cancer, to condoms, which we don't control because it's men who have to wear them—have some drawback," notes Linda Villarosa, author of *Body & Soul: The Black Woman's Guide to Physical Health and Emotional Well-Being* (HarperPerennial, $22). "It's a complex choice, and one that a woman must decide with her sexual partner." To help you with that choice, carve out some time so that you and your partner can assess the following snapshots of today's offerings. Then review the At-a-Glance Chart on page 237 and write down your impressions of how each option will work for the two of you. Check out the selection:

CONDOMS

Male and female condoms are the only form of birth control that provides protection against pregnancy and sexually transmitted diseases. Male condoms, made out of latex (thin rubber), are placed on an erect penis prior to intercourse. Female condoms, made out of a thin polyurethane sheath, are inserted into the woman's vagina before intercourse. Both types of condoms prevent sperm from entering the cervix by providing barrier protection. Fibroid sufferers shouldn't have any problems with either of these methods as long as each is used correctly.

THE PILL

The pill prevents conception by suppressing ovulation, thickening the cervical mucus to block sperm, and thinning out the endometrial lining to stop implantation of the fertilized egg. It's able to do this by distributing synthetic hormones through a small tablet that users take daily for twenty-one or twenty-eight days. The pill comes in two forms: birth control pills, which are combined oral contraceptives, or minipills which contain only progestin as a contraceptive agent. For maximum effectiveness, the pill should be taken the same time each day as a routine.

Views regarding whether or not you should take birth control pills if you've had trouble with fibroids are mixed. Nelson H. Stringer, author of *Uterine Fibroids: What Every Woman Should Know*, insists that "women who have had fibroids removed by myomectomy should not use birth control pills." He says that since birth control pills contain estrogen, the agent that causes fibroids to grow, women who use them will find an increase in the size of their myomas.

Other physicians disagree. "Having fibroids is not a good reason to avoid birth control pills," cautions Henderson. "Those contraceptives that are not hormonal will have the least effect on fibroids." Doctors that share Henderson's view say birth control pills containing a low dose of estrogen should not greatly affect the growth of myomas and they have no problem prescribing birth control pills to fibroid patients, so you may be offered them as a primary option. Adds Henderson, "Birth control pills have a lot of benefits other than preventing pregnancy (such as lower incidence of anemia related to bleeding and a lower incidence of ovarian cancer, for example). . . . Women with fibroids tend to feel the same as women who do not have them."

For me, the use of birth control pills was borderline disaster. Doctors prescribed them to help regulate my erratic periods and manage the excessive bleeding that was being caused by the fibroids. No success! The effectiveness of the treatment was temporary at best. The bleeding would stop for a few days and then return in full force. And what did the doctor do to combat this? Tell me to increase my daily intake by raising the number and dosage of the birth control pills. As a result, my fibroids were ballooning at a fast rate. At each visit, the size of them would multiply.

I contacted my cousin Debra, the one who works as a nurse practitioner, for help and she sent me to Dr. F. The Manhattan-based gynecologist was one of the few highly acclaimed fertility specialists that accepted insurance coverage. All of the other high-end experts preferred cash.

To my dismay, Dr. F was convinced that the bleeding would stop if he just matched me up with the right birth control pill. Give me a break; that's what the other eight doctors had tried to do, and they weren't even specialists. By that time, I was frustrated and tired of bleeding all over everything. So I wrote Dr. F a long letter outlining my horrid experiences and nearly begged him for surgery. He complied, even though he felt that you shouldn't have surgery unless you're trying to conceive. No, I wasn't trying to get pregnant, but I was miserable and I didn't know what else to do. In August 1997, I had a myolysis. The procedure, which was relatively new at the time, did shrink the fibroids by blocking their blood supply and the bleeding stopped—for about two years. As it turned out, a myolysis is about the worst procedure you can get if you want to have children because it weakens the uterus, but we didn't know that then. And even if we did, what choice did I have? The birth control pills weren't working.

SPERMICIDES

Spermicides, which come in the form of foam, jellies, or supposi-tories, must be inserted into the vagina fifteen minutes prior to in-tercourse. Typically used along with another contraception such as a diaphragm, condom, or cervical cap, spermicides work by blocking the entrance of the cervix and killing sperm on contact. Although the prod-ucts are widely available and easy to find, 30 percent of the couples that use spermicides as their only contraceptive experience an unplanned pregnancy within one year of use.

IUD (INTRAUTERINE DEVICE)

An IUD is a pregnancy prevention apparatus that is inserted into the womb by a doctor. Currently, there are two types of IUDs on the market in the United States. The Paragard Copper T 380A, which re-leases copper, can stay in place for ten years, and the Progestasert Pro-gesterone T, which releases progesterone (a form of progestin), requires replacement every year.

The IUD, which must be implanted by a physician, can be used by women with fibroids in some instances. However, "if you have a sub-

mucous myoma, an IUD can irritate it causing bleeding or spotting,"
cautions Cyril Spann, M.D., associate professor of OB/GYN at Emory
University. Although the IUD declined in popularity in the 1970s due
to a scare surrounding the Dalkon Shield, an IUD that was associated
with twelve deaths due to miscarriage-related infections, the two other
IUDs that remain on the market are probably the most popularly used
types of birth control worldwide.

DEPO-PROVERA

Depo-Provera, an injection that has been approved for contraceptive use in the United States since 1992, prevents ovulation for at least
fourteen weeks. The technique inhibiting ovulation is the same used by
birth control pills. Like birth control pills, Depo-Provera has been
found to reduce the risk of developing breast cancer. Users of Depo-
Provera also had a lower incidence of uterine cancer than nonusers.
According to experts, Depo-Provera's effectiveness is not affected by
antibiotics, so you won't have to worry about becoming pregnant should
you need to take antibiotics. In addition, Depo-Provera injections do
not contain estrogen, so you won't suffer the same side effects as birth
control users.

On the flip side, you may be concerned about the unpredictable
changes that may occur in your menstrual cycle. Women using Depo-
Provera may initially experience (in the first three months) irregular
bleeding or spotting over several days. Further, around half of women
using Depo-Provera for one year don't have a period at all—which is
viewed as a benefit by some and cause for alarm by others. You should
also know that the National Black Women's Health Project (NBWHP)
and other health organizations such as the National Women's Health
Network do not support the use of Depo-Provera because of the side
effects associated with this method according to Villarosa's book.

NORPLANT

The Norplant (subdermal implant) consists of six silicon capsules
that are inserted through a small incision under the skin in an arc for-
mation. The capsules release steady daily doses of the synthetic hor-

mone progestin to prevent conception. This method prevents pregnancy in a variety of ways. It suppresses ovulation and alters the cervical mucus so that migrating sperm are never able to reach the womb. Beyond that, the Norplant suppresses the development and growth of the lining of the uterus (endometrium), which hinders the egg from implanting in the womb. As you might imagine, this method is nearly 100 percent effective and does not rely on the user for effectiveness. There's no way you could mess this one up.

As with any other contraceptive method, the Norplant has side effects. Irregular menstrual bleeding, which usually occurs around the first three to six months, tops the list. Other complaints may include amenorrhea (temporary absence of the menstrual cycles), slight weight gain or loss, headaches, acne, breast discharge, transient ovarian cysts, enlarged ovaries, moodiness, vaginal discharge, dizziness, hair loss, itching, nausea, and nervousness. But many of these are uncommon and the relationship between these symptoms and the Norplant has not been confirmed. It's also been found that the Norplant is less effective in heavier women, those weighing 150 pounds or more.[2] "This is an important factor for Black Women to note, since we have so many large sisters in our community," insists Villarosa. She also advises that you consult a physician if you experience heavy vaginal bleeding, missed periods, arm pain, intense lower abdominal pain, pus or bleeding from the insertion spot, or if an implant appears to be coming out.

The Norplant is worry-free contraception for women who know they don't want to conceive for at least another five years (three years with the Norplant 2) and don't want to worry about remembering to take a pill on a regular basis. Plus, the Norplant doesn't contain estrogen, and that's a big plus for women with fibroids. Further, the insertion process takes all of five to ten minutes, while the removal process takes thirty minutes at the most.

DIAPHRAGM

The diaphragm, a flexible domelike apparatus, has to be fitted by a physician. It is inserted in the vagina along with spermicide prior to intercourse so that it covers the cervix, or neck of the womb. Be aware that the diaphragm must remain in place for at least six hours following intercourse but not for more than twenty-four hours. If you have sex more than once while wearing the diaphragm, you can leave it in place and add more spermicide by using a small plastic plunger. You can pick up the spermicide at any drugstore and you don't need a prescription.

You need to be refitted if the size of your cervix changes due to weight gain of ten pounds or more, pregnancy, an abortion, a miscarriage, or pelvic surgery. For the best protection, use the diaphragm along with a condom.

CERVICAL CAP

The cervical cap operates exactly as it sounds. Your gynecologist will fit you for a small soft rubber cup that you put into the vagina to fit over your cervix or neck of the womb prior to a sexual encounter. Prior to inserting it in your vagina, you should place nonoxynol-9 spermicide inside the cap to kill any sperm that wiggles its way pass the barrier. Although the cap is smaller than the diaphragm, it can also be more difficult to insert. You can leave the cap in position for forty-eight hours. It comes in several different sizes that can be purchased at drugstores without a prescription.

For further protection and to avoid sexually transmitted diseases, use the cervical cap with a condom. Also, get refitted if the size of your uterus changes, which can happen in response to weight gain, pregnancy, an abortion, a miscarriage, or pelvic surgery. In addition, contact your physician immediately if you start to show symptoms such as fever, vomiting, muscle pain, diarrhea, a rash, or dizziness because these signs could indicate toxic shock syndrome (TSS).

FEMALE STERILIZATION

Sis, if you're considering having a tubal ligation or a tubectomy (blocking of the fallopian tubes), think again. Female sterilization is permanent, so that means you'll never be able to have children in the future—even if you meet Mr. Wonderful in the next three months. If that's not an issue for you and you decide to go ahead, you'll obtain membership to a very popular club—sterilization is the world's most widely used contraceptive.

The outpatient surgery is typically performed under general anesthesia. It involves tying, cutting, or blocking the fallopian tubes so that your eggs will no longer be able to access the womb. Getting a highly skilled surgeon is key. Also, remember that you'll still have your period, but you don't have to worry about becoming pregnant ever again.

MALE STERILIZATION

Ever thought of leaving the responsibility of birth control in the hands of your lover? If you and the man in your life have no intentions of having children, the two of you should consider a vasectomy. This male surgical procedure promotes blockage of the vas deferens so that the sperm never merges with the semen. Following a vasectomy, sperm is absorbed in the body. The one-time procedure is safe, simple, and highly effective. It requires no follow-up medical care and its benefits outweigh those of female sterilization. For example, a vasectomy is performed in a doctor's office under local anesthesia and is simpler and less expensive than female sterilization.

One of the biggest problems with male sterilization is the male perception that a vasectomy is an assault on one's manhood. A vasectomy is not castration; the physician does not remove any glands or organs. The production of hormones and sperm never stops. In addition, the male continues to maintain an erection and there is little effect on his ejaculation, since only 5 percent of this fluid is sperm. In fact, the biggest difference the male may experience after a vasectomy is a new freedom that comes with not having to worry about impregnating someone.

On the flip side, two 1993 studies have found that a vasectomy may increase a man's risk of developing prostate cancer. This finding is particularly significant to African Americans since black men are more at risk for this type of cancer than their white counterparts.[3]

NATURAL FAMILY PLANNING

If you know your body, then you should be able to pinpoint that time when you're ovulating—that's the window of opportunity for an anxious sperm. This practice is also referred to as "fertility awareness" or "periodic abstinence." If you're relying on this method, it means you and your honey must refrain from having sex on the days when you are most likely to become pregnant unless you're using another form of birth control. The prime time for pregnancy typically ranges from seven days before you ovulate (release an egg) until three days following ovulation.

How do you know when you're ovulating? Your body will give off clues such as a reduced body temperature and marked changes in your vaginal mucus. If you still can't tell when you're ovulating, you can buy an ovulation kit (which is pretty costly) at the drugstore or ask your doctor for further instruction.

THE CHOICE IS YOURS

"The more you know about each type of contraceptive and the better you understand your own body, the easier the choice will be," points out Linda Villarosa in her book *Body and Soul: The Black Woman's Guide to Physical Health and Emotional Well-Being* (HarperPerennial, $22). No matter what method you choose, it won't do you any good unless you use it carefully, correctly, and consistently. Then, once you choose a birth control method that meets your needs, get an appointment with a GYN or hotfoot it to the nearest drugstore. Fibroids have been interfering with your romance long enough; it's time to get your groove on.

		Birth Control Choices			
Birth Control Method	Pros	Cons	Price	Where do I get this from?	How do I think this will work for me? (fill in)
Cervical Cap	You control it. Can be inserted in advance. Good for women who have infrequent intercourse. Easy to use. No long-term side effects.	Limited availability. Limited protection against STDs. Must be fitted by health professional. Could increase risk of infection of normal Pap smears.	Cap costs $30 each. Doctor visit for fitting at least $100.	Cervical Cap Ltd. 430 Monterey Ave., Suite 1B Los Gatos, CA 95030 408-395-2100	
Male Condom	Widely available. Inexpensive. Best prevention against STDs. No long-term side effects.	Must rely on male for proper use. Disrupts sexual continuity. Could be used incorrectly, has high failure rate. Breakage is common.	$1 each. Can get free from a clinic.	Any drugstore or corner store	
Female Condom	You control proper use. Will be widely available and easy to find. Failure rate is low if properly used. More resistant	Disrupts sexual continuity. Difficult to insert. Some say they are unattractive and awkward. Cost twice as much as male condom.	$2.50 each	Not widely available yet but you should be able to purchase at the same place as male condom.	

Birth Control Method	Pros	Cons	Price	Where do I get this from?	How do I think this will work for me? (fill in)
	to tears than male condom. Prevents spread of STDs. No long-term side effects.				
Depo-Provera The Shot	Highly Effective Easy to use. May reduce anemia.	Regular visits to a GYN for injections. Fertility can be delayed for several months after use. Side effects aren't immediately reversible. Doesn't prevent STDs.	$25 to $30	At your gynecologist's office or health clinic.	
Diaphragm	Can be inserted up to six hours in advance of sexual activity. Inexpensive. Can last for at least two years if properly stored.	Must be fitted by health personnel. Could become dislodged during intercourse. Doesn't protect against STDs. Shouldn't be used by women prone to urinary tract infection.	Between $15 and $35, plus doctor visit fee.	Physician	
IUD Intrauterine Devices	Reversible Highly effective and easy to use.	Need health professional for insertion and removal.	$300 plus doctor visit fees.	Physician	

Birth Control Method	Pros	Cons	Price	Where do I get this from?	How do I think this will work for me? (fill in)
	Can be inserted after a woman gives birth or has an abortion. Can be inserted after unprotected sex to prevent conception.	Insertion may hurt. Can cause irregular bleeding and cramping. In rare cases can perforate uterus. May increase risk of developing pelvic inflammatory disease (PID). Can get an infection during time of insertion.			
Natural Family Planning	No medical personnel required. No side effects. Causes you to learn about your body. Increases chances of becoming pregnant when you want to because woman understands her body.	High failure rate. Meticulous record keeping is required. Medical conditions can alter accuracy of readings. Doesn't protect against STDs.	It's free.	For information on ovulation method, write to: Family of the Americas Foundation PO Box 1170 Dunkirk, MD 20754-1170 800-443-3395 301-627-3346 Read: Your Ferility Signals: Using Them to Achieve or Avoid Pregnancy	

Birth Control Method	Pros	Cons	Price	Where do I get this from?	How do I think this will work for me? (fill in)
				Naturally by Merryl Winstein	
Norplant	Highly effective Easy to use. Good for long-term protection. May reduce anemia.	Causes irregular bleeding. Long list of possible side effects. High costs on front end. More effective for women under 150 pounds. Must be removed by medical professional. May cause scarring such as keloids.	$400–600 for capsules and procedure	Physician	
The pill	You control its use. Highly effective. Protects against ovarian and uterine cancer as well as benign cysts on the ovaries and breasts. Reduces risk of pelvic infections and ectopic preg-	Requires daily pill taking for effectiveness. You need a prescription. Could increase blood clots in women who smoke. May cause weight gain, tender breasts, and spotting between periods. Doesn't protect against STDs. Not uniformly	$10–30 plus doctor fee visits.	Drugstore with prescription from your doctor.	

Birth Control Method	Pros	Cons	Price	Where do I get this from?	How do I think this will work for me? (fill in)
	nancies. Regulates periods. Is taken daily at the same time.	recommended for women with fibroids.			
Spermicides	You control it. Widely available. Some protection against STDs. Doesn't have long-term side effects.	High rate of failure. May cause itching or burning. Must use close to the time of intercourse.	$4–12	Convenience and drugstores.	
Sterilization	You control it. Highly effective Little follow-up care needed. Cost is low since its protection is over long term. Good for women who don't want to bear children in the future.	Generally not reversible. High front-end costs. Requires skilled physician to perform surgery. Temporary discomfort from surgery. Doesn't protect against STDs.	$1,000–2,500	Get referral: Association of Voluntary Surgical Contraception 79 Madison Ave., 7th Floor New York, NY 10016 212-561-8000	
Vasectomy for male	Highly effective. Performed with local	Generally not reversible. Must rely on male for honesty.	$250–500	For referrals: Association of Voluntary Surgical	

Birth Control Method	Pros	Cons	Price	Where do I get this from?	How do I think this will work for me? (fill in)
	anesthesia. Little follow-up care required. Good if you don't want children in the future.	Male may experience discomfort following surgery. Doesn't protect against STDs.		Contraception 79 Madison Ave., 7th Floor New York, NY 10016 212-561-8000	
Withdrawal	Requires no medical professional.	High failure rate. Must rely on male. Doesn't protect against STDs. Interferes with lovemaking.	Free	When, how, and if this technique is used is up to you and your partner.	

Two new birth control methods are the vaginal ring and the contraceptive patch. "You leave the ring inside for three weeks and take it out for a week to have your period. As for the patch, you wear a new one for three weeks and then break for your period," explains Paula McKenzie, M.D., a Virginia-based gynecologist. "With these two advances in technology, women will have more choices in effective, convenient contraceptive methods."

15 | Making Connections

Building a Support Team You Can Count On

It's really been a challenge for me. But the support of family and friends made it easier. Whether you're married or not, if you have a partner that's supportive, they're invaluable. My husband Kyle has been exceptional.

Dealing with a fibroid, the baby, my worries and fears about my being over thirty-five has put a whole new perspective on things. And on top of everything, I was really concerned about birth defects. So I know firsthand that any woman having a baby needs support. Listen up, ladies, you need SUPPORT!

If you can't get it from family or friends, I suggest going to a church or outreach center or even an unwed mother facility. Just because you're not financially challenged doesn't mean you don't need support.

—Diantha Greenidge, Age 35, Accounting Manager

I'll never forget the first time I read *In the Company of My Sisters: Black Women and Self-Esteem* (Plume, $11) by Julia Boyd. It was a book that showcased how a group of African American women were able to transform their lives through an informal support group. Essentially, these sisters just sat around chatting about the "going ons" and "going offs" in their lives. But somehow these women were able to learn from one another and develop into better human beings.

That book changed my life. Until then, I thought it was my utmost duty to keep my "personal stuff" in the confines of my closet. Like other "strong" black women, I was taught to inhale my anger, repress my joy, and handle my business. After all, as long as I could get up and make it on time to my J-O-B, did anything else matter?

Of course it did. And Julia Boyd, through her words and wisdom, showed me that there were other women who were feeling just as empty as I had been feeling. There were women, black women, who weren't afraid to bare their souls for the sake of physical and mental healing. It was truly a revelation—thanks, girlfriend.

As a result of my newfound freedom—yes, being able to share with others is truly liberating—my friend Colette and I developed a support group for minority women. It is called Professional Women of Color (PWC), a nonprofit organization that sponsors workshops, seminars, and group discussions to help women of color balance their personal and professional lives. On a monthly basis, about forty women come together to network and just "kick it." These ladies are at various educational and professional levels and they represent a variety of organizations. Still, they all have three things in common: they have a burning desire to listen, understand, and share. So as you might imagine, aside from exchanging essential information for self-development, our meetings are filled with "Girl, you know exactly how I feel." Or "Sis, that's the same thing that happened to me." Together we learn that black women are even stronger when they make a commitment to support the betterment of the sisterhood.

So what does PWC (212-714-7190) have to do with fibroids? A few years ago, PWC sponsored a standing-room-only health conference at the Sister-to-Sister Uptown bookstore (212-862-3680) in Harlem. Although it was a general seminar about women's reproductive health, the subject of fibroids was a major topic of discussion. It's no wonder, the majority of the sisters in the room were having some challenges with them and they wanted answers. Of course our guest physicians could only offer some suggestions because they didn't have all of the answers back then—and as you know, there's more research that needs to be done today. Still, the sentiments expressed at the seminar illustrated just how prevalent fibroids are among African American women. It also gave me access to a long list of sisterfriends whom I could call when my fibroids were getting the best of me. Through PWC I was able to tap into a circle of friends that provided a safe environment for me to express my feelings without the fear of repercussion.

But your support doesn't have to be a list of members from an official organization or a group of close girlfriends. Get support where you can find it. Enlist both men and women in your support group by chatting with them in person (how about lunch?), by telephone, online, or through e-mails. Maintaining some type of support system is essential to your mental and physical well-being because networking can foster important links to doctors, support groups, health remedies, and insights on medical alternatives. Rely on members of your support team to accompany you to your doctor visits so you can feel more relaxed during these times as you prepare a list of questions for your gynecologist. If the two of you are comfortable and your physician allows it, you may have your buddy present while you're being examined or talking to your doctor afterward. Take it from me, things are never as bad as they seem once you allow others to weigh in on the situation. And if that isn't enough motivation for you to seek support, then just find comfort in knowing that sharing our concerns with one another is all a part of the master plan. When I was going through my challenges with fibroids in the midst of a terrible breakup of a five-year relationship, my cousin, Pam, sent me a card that read: "God never meant for us to handle challenges alone. That's why he gave us other people." Need I say more?

There are connections all around you. Here's how you can make a link:

TALK TO MOM

My mother (and father, for that matter) was invaluable during my fibroid saga and I was sorry that I hadn't allowed her to help me sooner. After all, that's what parents are for—really! Don't make the same mistake I did; let your mom (or dad) help you in your time of need.

To make the mom-daughter connection, shop 'til both of you drop. Take some time out for an afternoon tea. Or sneak into her sleeping chambers a few minutes before she drifts off to slumber. Do whatever, whenever, to develop the appropriate strategy and setting that will enable you to invite your mother (or mother figure) to aid in your healing. Regardless of how the two of you relate today—whether it's like close sisters or distant strangers—you can use the subject of fibroids to build a more fulfilling relationship.

How? For one thing, find out how much she knows about the prevalence of fibroids among your female relatives. Although there is no concrete evidence to prove that fibroids run in families, "at least 7 out of 10 patients have family members such as a mother, daughter, or sister with fibroids," cites diagnostic interventional radiologist Henry J. Krebs, III, M.D. Your mother may be able to tell you how she dealt with her fibroids or at least point you in the direction of other sufferers so they can offer their insights. In addition, don't make any assumptions about your mother's fibroid-fighting knowledge. Ask her everything you want to know and rely on her for comfort during the whole ordeal. The depths of her strength and support may surprise you. In addition, you may find that not only does Mom know best, she loves best too.

ASK ABOUT THE HISTORY OF FIBROIDS IN YOUR FAMILY

Talking to Mom is a great starting point, but you still need to make other family connections to get the full picture. The first connection should be made with you. It's essential that you know and record your medical, social, and family history so that you can spot patterns, track changes in your own medical developments, serve as a knowledgeable participant in your treatment, and be a resource to other members of your family. The information should be kept in a safe place that is easily accessible to family members should you be in an emergency situation. And don't limit your information gathering to fibroids—you need a full perspective of your medical history for true healing.

As a first step, consider Dr. Melody T. McCloud's guide *The Health Diary for Women of Color: Your Personal Log* (New Life Publishing, $9.95). It contains a host of thought-provoking questions and features a section on reproductive health that focuses on fibroid tumors as well as other gynecological issues. This information may prove priceless whenever you need to make important decisions about your health. "So many conditions women suffer from 'run in the family'; or, due to similar lifestyle tendencies, continue to reoccur generation after generation. By making a deliberate effort to review the history of one's family members', and one's own personal medical history and lifestyle, certain facts will become clear," notes McCloud.

But how do you get the information gathering going? McCloud says the process can be fun if you make it a family affair that includes your grandparents, mother, father, and siblings as well as other relatives. Imagine exchanging health history, habits, and facts over a healthy soul food Sunday dinner. This will enable all of you to come to terms with some of the bad habits you share and develop strategies for improvements. It will also provide the family with an opportunity to reminisce over the good things too—"remember Aunt Jane, who lived to 103 years old?" Sis, there's no stronger support system than the ties that bind family.

JOIN A SUPPORT GROUP

Hey you, have you ever had the feeling that you were in a situation that only a fellow sisterfriend could understand? You're not alone; it's estimated that between seven and twelve million Americans, mostly women, are active in self-help groups.[1] African American women, especially, can use self-help groups (mutual support groups) as tools to confront issues related to being black and female in America as well as collectively assess statistical data to pinpoint primary issues in the community. Self-help groups provide one more option that you can use as a part of your larger support system.

Before joining any group, do your research. Sit in on a meeting and think about what you want the group to help you accomplish, as well as whether or not you have time to dedicate to the group's meetings and activities. Then determine if the meeting location(s), time of day, membership fees and costs, culture, leadership, and member responsibilities are in alignment with your own values. If not, find another group, because you should never join any group to try to change it. Also understand that you won't gain any benefits unless you actively participate. Organizations need membership support to thrive and grow. If you find that you're only serving as a bystander or critic, do everyone a favor and bow out.

START A SUPPORT GROUP OF YOUR OWN

You don't have to start a formal nonprofit organization to be effective. You can just invite a few friends over to your house and ask them to bring guests. Your only requirement for admittance is that they be willing to share whatever experiences they've had with fibroids with the rest of the group. You might find that some of your guests have a lot in common or maybe they'll all gain some insight and a new outlook. Whatever the case, you're sure to have a grand time because there's no better gathering than the sisterfriend collective.

Debrena Jackson Gandy, author of *All The Joy You Can Stand*

(Crown, $22), agrees. "Developing intimate connections with other sisters replenishes my spirit, grounds me, and energizes me like nothing else can," she writes. To ensure an intimate setting that's conducive to an open honest exchange, Jackson Gandy suggests that you invite your girlfriends to your home rather than some public place like a restaurant. For her girlfriends, Jackson Gandy hosts an annual pamper party where she provides the ladies with a unique relaxation gift each year. Prior treats include hand massages, feet washing, and evening tea. For her thirty-second birthday, Jackson Gandy hosted a pajama party. Any of these ideas or ones that you develop can be used as the backdrop for your gathering. "When we gather with other sistahs in the spirit of nonjudgment, authenticity, acceptance, love, and truth telling, *healing happens*," adds Jackson Gandy.

WORK THE WEB

Maybe you can go online to manage nearly every aspect of your life. Or maybe you rarely surf the net. Whatever the case, don't overlook the Internet as an area that can provide support for your fibroids. According to Johanna Skilling, "virtual relationships that develop online can feel just as strong, or stronger, than some of our 'real life' encounters. After all there's another human being out there, typing away on her keyboard, thinking of you."

So type "fibroid" in any search engine and you're sure to get a long list of related sites. Many of these links have message boards or chat rooms that enable you to exchange information with other fibroid sufferers. There are even some sites that pass your questions on to practicing gynecologists.

Still, don't take everything you read on the Internet as gospel. Consider the people or organization that is affiliated with the site. For instance, if the organization favors "natural remedies," that information will probably be the most prevalent on the site. Check the dates of postings to ensure that the information you're reading is accurate. Recent postings indicate that there is someone actively managing the site. Also, check out the site for elements such as neatness, design, and grammar. If the site's sponsors don't even bother to run a spell check, that shows a lack of interest in the site's content and you shouldn't consider the site very reliable.

E-MAIL

When my AOL account sounded that I had mail, I never dreamed it would have such valuable information. It all started with feedback from one of my online buddies—you see the power of sharing—who connected me with an African American holistic practitioner based in South Africa to coach me through my fibroid saga. When I sent my e-mail, detailing the events of my fibroid experience and asking for advice on how I could decide about my upcoming surgery, I had no idea what would become of it. But the results well exceeded my wildest expectations.

Dr. Yvonne Paris-Fergerson zapped over a complete eating regimen for me as well as a host of holistic remedies to treat my complaints. She also gave me the contact information for another fibroid sufferer that was based here in New York, Arlene. Initially Arlene and I served to support each other through our various fibroid challenges, but as time passed we also developed a very fulfilling friendship. We party together, vacation together, and help each other with issues that don't have anything to do with fibroids. Who knew?

WRITE TO A MAGAZINE

I'd start with health, African American, or women's magazines, but you may find other ones that are receptive to covering fibroids if they haven't recently run a story on them or if you can offer a unique angle for future coverage. A basic way to get support from magazines is to send in an inquiry for the publication's "question and answer" column. Here the editors turn to experts that can address your question directly. Typically they feature the writer's name, city, and state but you can request that these be withheld for confidentiality. The important thing is that you can get information from the same experts that magazine editors use as resources just by asking a question. Magazines are great sources of information because their editorial content is typically based on the latest research.

You may also opt to pitch an idea for a small article or a feature story. Some of the best magazine articles are developed from ideas submitted by the publication's readers, so don't be afraid to ask them to publish a story on fibroids if you think the topic fits into their overall mission. Just be aware that magazine editors (the people who make the decisions about what articles run in the publication) need to be convinced that the approach you suggest will offer a different perspective than competitor publications. Editors also don't like to revisit a topic within the same two-year period unless it's particularly important or unique. So you may want to browse the magazine's archives on their web site to see if they've recently done articles on fibroids. Even if they have, you can still pitch the idea if you feel it offers new information that will be useful to the publication's readers. After receiving your query letter (a one-page statement of your idea and why you think it's an important topic for the magazine), they may want to feature you as one of the subjects of the story. Further, if you've always wanted to try your hand at writing, your fibroid saga may enable you to parlay some freelance opportunities. But you'll never know what lies ahead unless you check the publication's masthead (list of employees and titles in the front of the magazine) or web site to determine who should get your inquiry letter or e-mail and put pen to paper.

CALL ON A FRIEND

When my friend told me that she was having problems with her fibroids, I took to the Internet and started searching for solutions. At first, I didn't quite know what I was looking for. The only thing I knew was that my buddy looked about five months pregnant and she fingered fibroids as the prime suspect. Soon, however, my inquiries returned loads of results and I repackaged this information to send to my friend. Although I admitted that I didn't know the first thing about what she was dealing with, I did feel that her condition—from what I saw—had gotten way out of hand. It was time for her to act. Ultimately she took my advice and had a myomectomy. Now she raves about her petite tummy and says she owes it all to me.
—Jonathan Blakley, 32, Newsman

I don't know what would have happened to me if Jonathan hadn't interceded when he did. Prior to his interference (as I initially called it), I didn't have a life. Outside of work, I never went outside because it was to the point where I could have a bleeding spell at any minute. During that "time of the month" I covered the floors, the furniture, and the bed with newspaper and towels and wore Depends (adult diapers) for added protection—but none of these things prevented the accidents. In addition, my abdomen was growing at an alarming rate; it was the size of a twenty-week pregnancy (five months) and still growing. To conceal it and still fit into my clothes, I started wearing several pairs of girdle undergarments—this was a painful, uncomfortable experience. So when my gynecologist stated in no uncertain terms that I needed a myomectomy and scheduled it in four weeks, I reluctantly agreed.

But agreeing verbally was the easy part; mentally, I was a wreck. My fear about a possible hysterectomy (an outcome that could occur in the event of an emergency) overwhelmed me. Even the slightest chance of a mishap was more than I was willing to risk, so I chickened out three days prior to the surgery. Next, I went into denial mode convincing myself that things weren't as bad as they seemed. In addition, I tripled my visits to church and stepped up my praying habits. This allowed me to believe (at least on some level) that my fibroids would just magically disappear due to the support of the praying pastor and congregation. The evidence, however, showed that things were getting progressively worse.

Jonathan caught a glimpse of my enlarged belly during a visit when I was walking around the house girdle-free in my casual gear. Although he didn't express it at the time of the visit, he was alarmed. On the following Monday, he sent me an e-mail emphasizing the importance of finding a surgeon who could help me reclaim my life. He begged me to overcome my fears so I could gain the courage to move forward. Somehow, he also helped me understand that I was more than a uterus and two fallopian tubes. This realization gave me the strength to have the surgery on August 17—one day after Jonathan's birthday. It was one of the best decisions I ever made, and I don't know if I would have made that decision without Jonathan's support.

Without a doubt, strong friendships made my fibroid experience a little more bearable. One of my longtime girlfriends, Josette, listened to my dilemma day in and day out and even put some of the calls on her long-distance bill. Karima shared some of her healing techniques with me and connected me with other people that she knew had fibroids so we could exchange information. Yudelka kept her research antennas up and called me when she heard anything about the subject of fibroids. And then there were those friends who just shared a kind word or sent out special prayers. All of their support was truly invaluable.

I encourage you to allow some of your friends, whether they be male or female, to help you in whatever way they can. If they don't know what fibroids are, explain it to them or let them read about it. Even if you're uncomfortable providing them with the specific details about your problem, you can still allow them to lend a hand. Try asking them to give you a lift to the doctor's office, keep you busy while you wait for test results, or pick up some extra items for you while they're at the grocery store. Use your fibroids as an excuse to allow your friends to express their love for you—it's allowed.

CREATE A WELLNESS TEAM

Deal with your fibroids by establishing a position of strength, advises holistic practitioner Queen Afua. She suggests that fibroid sufferers get a wealth of well-rounded advice from various professionals including a holistic health practitioner, acupuncturist, herbalist, and a holistic OB/GYN. Also, turn to various sources for other contacts in the health care industry. Women who have successfully been healed from their fibroids should also be on your team. Adds Queen Afua, once you have gathered support and knowledge from these various members of your wellness team and maintained a prayerful state, then you can experience your healing in a more intelligent manner.

SEEK PROFESSIONAL COUNSELING

Sometimes a problem, or at least our perception of a problem, requires insight from a trained mental health expert such as a psychiatrist or therapist. Seeking advice from a professional doesn't mean that you're mentally ill. You can also abandon the stereotype that says psychotherapy is only for crazy white people. Your decision to get help simply means that you are woman enough to recognize when a problem is beyond your tolerance level or understanding. According to Linda Villarosa, author of *Body & Soul: The Black Women's Guide to Physical Health and Emotional Well-Being* (HarperPerennial, $22), "Therapy can help you confront the emotional problems in your life and give you the tools to deal with them in a healthy, constructive manner."

No issue is too big or too small to call on a health professional for guidance. It's purely up to you. However, if you are having problems sleeping or are constantly depressed, nervous, suicidal, excessively tired, or unable to maintain your concentration, you should seek professional help. And you should never feel ashamed if you find you need counseling from an expert. You owe it to yourself to get the help you need to enhance your life.

Besides, talking out your concerns with an impartial person has undeniable benefits. The process enables you to gain new insight, organize your thoughts, understand yourself better, and help make the changes you need for healing. "For many black women, therapy can be a stimulus for growth, change and a reaffirmation of self-worth," notes Villarosa. "Counseling creates a space for you to drop the mask of being a 'strong Black woman' and gives you permission to express the truth about your fears, joys, worries, accomplishments, and frustrations."

Choose the Right Therapist

- **Determine how you're going to pay for the sessions.** Check with your human resources office to see if your firm will cover the cost of your visit(s). If not, evaluate your budget to come up with an amount that you can afford. Also look in your phone book for free counseling services or turn to a spiritual leader for advice.
- **Get a referral.** Contact your friends, family, or an employee referral service to get a therapist under your plan (if covered) and near your neighborhood.
- **Read up.** Go to your nearest library or bookstore for guidance on how you can select a therapist and what you can expect from the sessions. In addition, refer to "Healing with Therapy" (*Essence*, March 1992) and "A Guide to Psychotherapy (*Essence*, June 1989).
- **Choose someone you feel comfortable with.** Be honest about your needs. If you prefer an African American or female, then you might consider those factors when making your choice. You may want to consider Afrocentric Therapy, for example. With this spiritual approach, black women are taught that all of their experiences, whether they be good or bad, are blessings that lead to greater self-understanding. The important thing is to choose a practitioner that operates in your comfort zone.
- **Ask questions.** You should conduct an initial interview of the therapist or psychiatrist prior to participating in a formal session.

Write down a list of inquiries to get details on items such as the fees charged, cancellation policy, payment policies, the professional's educational background and years of experience in the field, the types of problems he or she typically treats, and the practitioner's experiences with dealing with African Americans (even if he or she is black).

- **Assess your counseling sessions.** Whether you've had one visit or several, determine whether you feel your counseling sessions work for you. As Villarosa notes, you always have the right to terminate therapy. "Don't stay with someone who is not meeting your needs," she adds.[2]

WHO IS ON YOUR SUPPORT TEAM?

Write down anyone who has already committed to helping you deal with your fibroid issues or some people that you'd like to enlist. Then set up some time to talk to them. Once they've shown their support, don't forget to say thank you.

Name	Phone number or contact info	How can they support me? (For example, provide additional information, listen to my concerns, tell me about their experiences)	When will we talk? (Write in a date)	Results

EPILOGUE

It's been more than a year since I had the myomectomy. And what a great year it has been! Aside from the huge keloid on my abdomen (I told you it was the size of a large, long pickle), there's almost no evidence that I had the surgery or the fibroids. I feel great. My periods have been almost pain-free, and they are lighter than ever. This year, I actually spent a night at someone else's home—that was almost unheard of prior to my surgery because I didn't want to run the risk of ruining their sheets, mattresses, or furniture. I'm also a lot less stressed and I eat healthier—although I do manage to sneak in a piece of chicken every now and then. But what do you expect? Now that I'm fibroid-free, I'm free to indulge in all of life's pleasures. And I love every single minute of it.

Speaking of love, I've managed to stir a little romance into the mix as well. Life's just a little sweeter when you have someone special to share it with, and that's the truth. My new honey bunny is named Jamie and he treats me like a queen—just like I deserve to be treated. You know I've already done the girlfriend/boyfriend thing and my last relationship was pure drama. (Remember the "brotha" that had a baby with someone else and lied about it for more than a year?) As a result, I decided to do things differently this time. Instead of falling in love, I walked into this relationship with both feet on the ground—that's the only way to do it! Our "thing" is based on truth, support, and consideration; all of these elements were missing in my last relationship.

Since cultivating a successful relationship takes work, I've decided to eliminate some of my extracurricular activities, reduce my hours at the office, and spend more time at home so I can work on taking care of me. I can't be any good to anyone else unless I do just that. They say balance is the key to life. I believe that and have found it to be an essential component of my newfound love and happiness.

But what do my decisions to make healthier choices, indulge in fulfilling relationships, and increase my me-time have to do with a book on fibroids? It's all part of the plan, girlfriend. My fibroids were trying to tell me something, and it took some drastic measures to force me to listen up. Loving myself was the first step toward healing, and I plan to continue on this path forever.

Now the question remains, what are your fibroids trying to tell you? Are you in an unfulfilling relationship? Have you denied yourself the benefit of life's simple pleasures? Are you stressed out? Are you caught up in living someone else's dream? Do you work in a job you hate? Are you bound by the clutches of self-pity or self-hatred? Is your spiritual house out of order? Your fibroids may be a manifestation of frustration. Sometimes our bodies sound the alarms to keep us from self-destructing. Watch the warnings and take heed, sis.

Consider yourself blessed. The next time your body chooses to catch your attention, it may be a lot worse than fibroids.

I wish you all the love and happiness your heart can take—squared! Good luck to you.

Peace and blessings,
Monique

GLOSSARY: TALK THAT TALK, GIRLFRIEND

Doctors like patients who are informed about their bodies and know the terms. They have a different respect for you when you come in prepared.
—Diantha Greenidge, Age 35, Accounting Manager

Acupuncture: A procedure in which needles are inserted at certain points of the body for relaxation or to treat certain conditions.

Adenomyosis: A noncancerous condition where the cells from the uterine lining start to grow inside the uterine muscle. (See Chapter 12: Copycat Syndromes.)

Adhesions: Scarring or small strands of fibrous tissue that cause the abnormal clinging and sticking of the surfaces inside the abdomen and pelvis, particularly in the uterus or fallopian tubes. Can occur from conditions such as endometriosis or as a result of certain surgical procedures like a myomectomy or myolysis.

Amenorrhea: Absence or cessation of periods. Primary amenorrhea occurs when a period does not start by age sixteen. Secondary amenorrhea is when a woman who is already menstruating and is not pregnant or going through menopause misses a period or periods.

Anemia: Results because of an insufficient amount of iron in the blood, an insufficient amount of hemoglobin in the blood, or less than the normal number of red blood cells.

Benign: No cancer is present. Not malignant. A benign tumor may grow, but it does not penetrate surrounding areas or spread to other body parts.

Biopsy: A sample of tissue or cells is removed so a pathologist can examine it under a microscope to determine if cancer cells are present.

Blood cells: There are two types of blood cells: red blood cells carry oxygen to tissues in the body, and white blood cells fight infection by tackling germs. One drop of blood contains 200 million red cells and 400,000 white cells.

Blood count: A count of red and white blood cells.

Blood pressure: The amount of pressure put on the walls of the arteries and blood vessels when the heart contracts and relaxes.

Blood transfusion: When blood from an outside source is pumped through a patient's veins. When a fibroid sufferer bleeds to the point where her hemoglobin is below 6, she may need a blood transfusion.

Blood vessels: The tubes—veins, arteries, capillaries—that enable blood to circulate through the body.

Cancer: An abnormal accelerated overgrowth of cells that harms surrounding tissue.

Cancerous growths: When the cells begin to mass and invade surrounding tissues.

Cervical cancer: When cancer is present in the cervix. (See Chapter 12: Copycat Syndromes.)

Clitoris: Small female genital organ located in the upper area of the vulva, which may result in sexual excitement and orgasm when stimulated.

Colposcopy: A lighted slender optical instrument that is used to visually examine the cervix.

Conception: When the egg becomes fertilized and implants in the uterine wall.

Condom: There are two types of condoms. The female version is typically made of polyurethane and is inserted in the vagina prior to intercourse to prevent pregnancy. It provides limited protection against STDs (sexually transmitted diseases). The male condom is a thin latex (preferably) sheath that is put on an erect penis prior to intercourse to prevent pregnancy. Although the male condom is the most effective protection against STDs, it is still not absolute. (See Chapter 13: Oh Baby!)

Contraception: The use of devices or techniques to prevent pregnancy. (See Chapter 14: No Baby!)

Curettage: A scraping process that's used to collect tissue from the lining of the uterus for laboratory examination so a condition can be diagnosed. It's the "C" portion of D&C. (See Chapter 4: Decisions, Decisions, Decisions.)

Curette: The sharp instrument used to collect tissue from the uterine lining or to scrape skin lesions.

Cyst: A sac that is filled with diseased matter or fluid. (See Chapter 12: Copycat Syndromes.)

Cyst aspiration: The removal of the cyst contents for a laboratory assessment.

D&C: Acronym for *Dilation and Curettage.*

Degeneration: The painful process where the fibroid begins to die and disintegrate because it has outgrown its blood supply or lacks adequate levels of estrogen. The pain typically passes within twenty-four hours. You may have a pink or brown discharge.

Diaphragm: A flexible dome-shaped rubber device that's inserted into the vagina so it cups the cervix and prevents sperm from entering the uterus. (See Chapter 13: Oh Baby!)

Dilation and curettage (D&C): With this diagnostic procedure the cervix is stretched (dilation) so that a spoon-shaped instrument (curette) is inserted into the womb to collect a portion of the lining (endometrium) so that the sample can be assessed in a laboratory.

Dysmenorrhea: Intense abdominal cramps or pain associated with menstruation.

Dyspareunia: Difficult or painful sexual intercourse.

Ectopic pregnancy: A condition where a fertilized egg implants in the wrong place such as the fallopian tubes or the peritoneal cavity.

Embryo: A description of the fertilized egg from the time it implants until the eighth week after conception.

Endometrial ablation: This procedure, where the uterine lining is removed or destroyed, is an approach taken when a woman suffers from heavy bleeding but is not an adequate treatment for fibroids. With this technique, the breakdown of blood from the endometrium (inner layer of the uterus or uterine lining) decreases or completely stops. *Ablation* is a word that means the surgical removal or excision. (See Chapter 5: Doctor's "Can Do" List.)

Endometrial biopsy: This diagnostic technique, most often performed in a doctor's office, is used to obtain a sample of the lining of the uterus (the endometrium). It's typically performed to learn the cause of abnormal uterine bleeding, find out the cause of infertility, evaluate uterine infections, or measure the impact of certain medications. Risks include cramping, pain, vaginal bleeding, infection, and rarely injury to the uterus.

Endometrial hyperplasia: A condition where there is overgrowth of the cells in the lining of the uterus (endometrium). *Hyperplasia* means overgrowth.

Endometriosis: A condition where cells from the uterine lining start to grow in places outside of the womb such as the fallopian tubes, ovaries, and other areas in the pelvis. (See Chapter 12: Copycat Syndromes.)

Endometrium: The cells within the uterine lining that shed monthly in response to the hormonal changes that occur during the menstrual cycle.

Estrogen: The female hormone produced by the ovaries that stimulates the growth of the uterine lining. After the menstrual cycle stops, during menopause, the ovaries and fatty tissues in the body make estrogen in smaller amounts.

Estrogen replacement therapy (ERT): An estrogen supplement treatment plan for women who have had their ovaries removed or experienced menopause.

Exploratory laparotomy: Examining and viewing the contents of the abdomen through a surgical incision.

Fallopian tubes: The flexible internal tube that serves as a passageway for the egg (ovum) to pass through to the uterus.

Fertilization: The process when the sperm penetrates the egg.

Fibroid tumors: The term *fibroid* is a misnomer. These uterine tumors are benign, or noncancerous, growths in the womb. They may or may not cause symptoms and they occur more often in African American women.

General anesthesia: The use of medications to cause a sleeplike state to prevent pain during surgery.

Gestation: The time a fetus spends in the mother's womb. Gestation is typically thirty-nine weeks from conception to delivery.

Gonadotropin-releasing hormone agonist (GnRHa): Drugs that manage the pituitary gonadotropes resulting in low FSH and LH secretion.

Hormone replacement therapy (HRT): Hormone treatment using estrogen alone or estrogen combined with synthetic (progestin) or natural progesterones for women who have had both ovaries removed or have experienced menopause.

Hot flashes: A heated sensation that can quickly overtake a woman's body. Hot flashes may occur frequently or rarely and generally last a minute or two. They may be a side effect for women who are getting GnRHa treatments or undergoing menopause.

Hysterosalpingography: A special x-ray test that enables the physician to get an inside view of the uterus and fallopian tubes by injecting a small amount of fluid into these areas to detect abnormal changes in the size and shape of the uterus and fallopian tubes and identify blockages.

Hysteroscopy: Inspection of the uterus or cervix with a lighted instrument (hysteroscope) that is inserted in the cervix and cavity of the uterus.

Hysterotomy: A surgical incision through the wall of the uterus.

Hysterectomy: The surgical removal of the entire uterus, which may or may not include the cervix, fallopian tubes, and ovaries. If the uterus is removed without removing the cervix, the procedure is referred to as a subtotal hysterectomy. When the uterus and cervix are removed it's called a total hysterectomy. If the ovaries are removed along with the uterus, menopause occurs instantly. Otherwise, the ovaries typically stop producing estrogen and progesterone soon after a hysterectomy (apparently they need the uterus to continue estrogen production) or continue to produce hormones until menopause happens naturally.

Incontinence: A condition where there is the loss of urine control, usually due to weakened muscles. Some women have "stress incontinence" and leak urine when they laugh or cough. Other women have "urge incontinence" and can't hold their urine once they feel the need to urinate.

Infertility: A condition where there is a reduced ability or inability to conceive and have offspring. Infertility is also defined in specific terms as the failure to conceive after a year of regular well-timed intercourse without contraception.

Laparoscope: A slender lighted telescope used to view the pelvic organs or to perform surgery.

Laparoscopy: A surgical procedure where a small incision (cut) is made in the abdominal wall so that a laparoscope can be passed through to view the pelvic organs or perform surgery. (See Chapter 4: Decisions, Decisions, Decisions.)

Laparotomy: A surgical procedure where an incision is made in the abdomen. (See Chapter 5: Doctor's "Can Do" List.) The word *laparotomy* is derived from Greek roots *lapara* meaning "soft part of the body between the rib cage and the hips" and *tome* meaning "a cutting."

Leiomyoma: A benign tumor derived from smooth muscle. Also referred to as a fibromyoma or myoma. Although leiomyomas are commonly called fibroids, the term is a misnomer.

Leiomyosarcoma: A rare malignant tumor of smooth muscle.

Libido: Sexual urge or drive.

Ligation, tubal: A surgical clipping or blockage of the fallopian tubes to permanently prevent pregnancy.

LMP: Last menstrual period.

Lupron: An injectable GnRH-based drug that temporarily shuts down the menstrual cycle by turning off the ovaries' ability to produce estrogen and progesterone.

Malignant: Cancer is present and the abnormal overgrowth will tend to spread or invade other organs or tissues (metastasize).

Menarche: The start of the menses.

Menopause: Date of last menstrual period. The natural permanent conclusion of menstruation where periods have been absent for twelve months.

Menorrhagia (hypermenorrhea): Irregular heavy menstrual flow.

Menorrhea: A normal menstrual flow.

Menses: The menstrual flow.

Menstrual: Relating to menstruation.

Menstruation: The periodic discharge of blood that flows from the uterus through the vagina approximately every four weeks in response to hormones produced by the ovaries in women who are not pregnant and who are of reproductive age. Menstruation is also called menorrhea. The time during which menstruation happens is referred to as menses.

Metrorrhagia: Irregular uterine bleeding that occurs at times other than the menses; usually not excessive bleeding.

Morcellation: The process where a morcellator is used to remove the uterus along with the fibroid(s) by cutting the womb into tiny pieces when performing the classic abdominal serrated macro-morcellator hysterectomy (CASH) procedure. With this technique the cervix is salvaged because of the belief that the cervix is important to sexual pleasure.

Naturopathic medicine or naturopathy: treats patient using natural substances and recognizes that a patient's emotional, mental, and physical state must be addressed for overall healing. Practitioners don't just treat a problem but try to remedy the condition that caused the problem by incorporating conventional medicine as well as therapeutic alternatives such as homeopathy, herbs, diet management, hydrotherapy, exercise, physical therapy, massages, and counseling.

Ovaries: Two walnut-shaped organs of the female body that produce eggs, estrogen, progesterone, and other hormones. At menopause, ovaries stop producing eggs but still produce some hormones.

Ovum: Term refers to an egg that is housed in the female ovary. This egg, which is also called the sex cell or female gamete, combines with the male gamete (sperm) to form a zygote and this is where fertilization occurs.

Pelvic inflammatory disease (PID): A severe infection that affects the female reproductive system, particularly the structures above the cervix, which may result from sexually transmitted diseases such as gonorrhea or chlamydia.

Perimenopausal: The time—whether it be months or years—leading up to the last period that will occur in response to reduced hormonal levels. When your periods are lighter, shorter, and irregular, those may be signs that menopause is soon to come.

Peritoneum: The membrane that lines the abdominal cavity and encases the internal organs.

PMP: Previous menstrual period.

Polymenorrhea: A condition where uterine bleeding occurs in frequent but regular instances, typically in intervals of twenty-one days or less.

Progesterone: An ovary-produced hormone that maintains the uterine lining. Upon menopause, the body reduces its production of progesterone.

Red degeneration: A complication during pregnancy where the fibroid begins to outgrow its blood supply, commonly around twenty weeks. Red degeneration is painful, lasting anywhere from a few days to more than a week. You may also notice light bleeding, nausea, vomiting, and a low-grade fever. It's one of the most common complications that fibroids can cause during pregnancy but one study reported that it only affects one in ten women. (See Chapter 13: Oh Baby!)

Resectoscope: A thin telescope with an electrical wire loop or rollerball tip that is used to remove or destroy uterine tissue.

Tumors: A cluster of abnormal, overgrowing cells. They are not necessarily cancerous or dangerous. Tumors can be hollow (cystic) or solid and are subdivided into benign (noncancerous) and malignant (cancerous).

Ultrasound: A test that uses high-frequency sound waves that bounce off of tissues using special devices. The echoes are transformed into results that are called a sonogram. Ultrasound imaging, called ultrasonography, provides an inside view of soft tissues and body cavities, without invasive techniques. Ultrasounds are also used to examine a fetus during pregnancy.

Uterus: Also referred to as the womb. The hollow, pear-shaped organ is located in the female's lower abdomen between the bladder and the rectum; it houses a fetus during pregnancy or releases the wastes from a disintegrating lining if an egg is not fertilized. The upper part of the uterus is called the corpus; it's made up of two layers of tissue.

Vagina: The muscular canal, lined with mucous membrane, extends from the cervix to the outside of the female body. It's typically about six to seven inches in length, and includes two vaultlike structures, the anterior (front) vaginal fornix and the posterior (rear) vaginal fornix. The vagina contains numerous small glands that make vaginal secretions. The word *vagina* is derived from the Latin word meaning "a sheath or scabbard."

RESOURCES

Gynecological Issues

American Association of Gynecological Laparoscopists
13021 East Florence Avenue
Santa Fe Springs, CA 90670
800-554-AAGL

American Association of Sex Educators, Counselors, and Therapists
P.O. Box 5488
Richmond, VA 23220-0488
312-644-0828
E-mail: aasect@assect.org
www.aasect.org

American College of Obstetricians and Gynecologists
409 Twelve Street SW
Washington, DC 20024-2188
202-638-5577

American Medical Women's Association
801 North Fairfax, Suite 400
Alexandria, VA 22314
703-838-0500
www.amwa.org

American Society for Psychosomatic OB/GYN
409 Twelve Street SW
Washington, DC 20024-2188
202-863-2414 or 863-2516

American Society for Reproductive Medicine
1209 Montgomery Highway

Birmingham, AL 35216
205-978-5000

Boston's Women Health Book Collective
240-A Elm Street
Somerville, MA 02144
617-625-0271
A women's health nonprofit organization offering health information
through its Women's Health Information Center.

CHOICE
Concern for Health Options, Information, Care and Education
125 South 9th Street, Suite 603
Philadelphia, PA 19107
215-985-3355

Georgetown University Medical Center
www.dml.georgetown.edu/fibroids

HealthGate.com
www.healthgate.com

Hysterectomy Educational Resources Services (HERS)
610-667-7757

International Center for Research on Women
1717 Massachusetts Avenue NW, Suite 302
Washington, DC 20036
202-797-0007

International Women's Health Coalition
24 East 21st Street, Fifth Floor
New York, NY 10010
212-979-8500

The Mayo Clinic
www.mayohealth.org

National Black Women's Health Project
1237 Abernathy Boulevard
Atlanta, GA 30310
800-275-2947

National Medical Association
1012 Tenth Street, NW
Washington, DC 20001
202-347-1895

National Women's Health Information Center
www.4woman.gov

National Self-Help Clearinghouse
33 West 42nd Street
New York, NY 10036
212-840-1259
Provides referrals and self-help newsletter.

National Women's Health Network
1325 G Street, NW
Washington, DC 20005
202-347-1140
Provides information on a variety of health topics, including fibroids.

National Women's Health Network's Information and Clearinghouse
202-628-7814
Call for a complete report on fibroids.

ObGyn.net
www.obgyn.net
Designed by a group of obstetricians and gynecologists.

Planned Parenthood
810 Seventh Avenue
New York, NY 10019
212-603-4600

Sex Information and Education Council of the United States
130 West 42nd Street, Suite 350
New York, NY 10036
212-819-9770

Sunspire Health
Offers published resources on uterine fibroids. Also has information
on holistic treatments for fibroids.
sunspire@mindspring.com
www.voicesofwomen.com/sunspire/home.html
888-786-7747

The Women's Interactive Site
www.womens-health.cfom

Uterine Fibroids
Sponsored by Brigham and Women's Hospital in Boston
www.fibroids.net

Exercise

Aerobics and Fitness Association of America (AFAA)
15250 Ventura Boulevard, Suite 200
Sherman Oaks, CA 91403
800-233-4886
Answers inquiries regarding exercise safety and effectiveness. Also
offers certification in personal training and aerobics.

African American Association of Fitness Professionals
1507 East 53rd Street, Suite 495
Chicago, IL 60615
312-854-5843
Provides information and networking opportunities for African
American professionals. Publishes newsletter on a quarterly basis.

African American Athletic Association, Inc.
355 Lexington Avenue, 16th Floor
New York, NY 10017
212-953-3100

In 1990, Arthur Ashe founded this support, advocacy, and resource organization for the benefit of African American athletes.

Agency for Healthcare Research and Quality (AHRQ)
Publications Clearinghouse
PO Box 8547
Silver Springs, MD 20907
800-358-9295
www.ahrq.gov/clinic/utersumm.htm
Duke University Evidence-Based Practice Center (EPC) summary of *Management of Uterine Fibroids* is available.

Black Women in Sports Foundation
PO Box 2610
Philadelphia, PA 19130
215-763-6609
A nonprofit organization that encourages and promotes black women in sports.

The Melpomene Institute
1010 University Avenue
St. Paul, MN 55104
651-642-1951
Provides research, education, and publications to girls and women that links physical activity to health.

Women's Sports Foundation
Eisenhower Park
East Meadow, NY 11554
516-542-4700
800-227-3988
Provides general information and advocates women in sports.

Women of Color in Sports
Adrienne R. Lotson
10236 W. 96th, #A
Overland Park, KS 66212
913-541-1864
Supports women of color in the area of sports.

Support

Sisterfriends
www.Sisterfriends.com
Virtual community for women of color. Covers a variety of topics including health, music, relationships, spiritual, sports, fitness, and the arts.

Weight Management

Healthy Weight Network
402 South 14th Street
Hettinger, ND 58639
701-567-2646
www.healthweightnetwork.com

Overeaters Anonymous
505-891-2664
www.overeatersanonymous.org

Shape Up America!
www.shapeup.org
Former U.S. Surgeon General C. Everett Koop's national campaign to fight obesity.

Size Acceptance Web Site
www.bayarea.net/~/Fatfaq/size.html

Take Off Pounds Sensibly (TOPS)
800-932-8677
www.tops.org

Weight Control Information Network
1 WIN Way
Bethesda, MD 20892
301-984-7378
800-WIN-8098
www.niddk.nih.gov/health/nutrit/win.htm

Natural Medicine

American Holistic Medical Association
6728 Old McLean Village Drive
McLean, VA 22101
703-556-9728
703-556-9245
www.holisticmedicine.org
Organization acknowledges the relationship between the spirit, mind and body. Referral service.

American Association of Acupuncture and Oriental Medicine
4101 Lake Boone Trail, Suite 201
Raleigh, NC 27607
919-787-5191

American Association of Naturopathic Physicians
601 Valley Street, Suite 105
Seattle, WA 98109
206-298-0125

Dr. Judyth Reichenberg-Ullman
Dr. Robert Ullman
Naturopathy and Homeopathy
206-774-5599

Herb Research Foundation
1007 Pearl Street, Suite 200
Boulder, CO 80302
303-449-2265

National Women's Health Network
514 Tenth Street, NW, Suite 400
Washington, DC 20004

Naturopathy Online, *www.naturopathyonline.com/nature.htm*

Participate in Clinical Trials/Research on Fibroids

The Agency for Health Care Policy and Research (AHCPR)
P.O. Box 8547
Silver Spring, MD 20907
800-358-9295
410-381-3150 (outside U.S.)
http://www.ahcpr.gov

CenterWatch, Inc.
22 Thomson Place, 12F3
Boston, MA 02210-1212
800-765-9647
email: *cntrwatch@aol.com*
http://www.centerwatch.com.

More information on Lupron
TAP Pharmaceuticals Medical Services Department
800-622-2011
http://www.lupron.com

The National Lupron Victims Network
609-858-2131
http://www.voicenet.com/net

To File a Complaint
Contact your state medical board

To Check Board Certification
American Board of Medical Specialties (ABMS)
http://www.certifieddoctor.org

To Perform Background Checks
American Medical Association
515 N. State Street
Chicago, IL 60610
312-464-5199
http://www.ama-assn.org/

Medi-Net
888-275-6334
Company charges a fee for background checks.

Accreditation Council for Gynecologic Endoscopy
P.O. Box 610
Downey, CA 90241-0610
562-946-4435
http://www.aagl.com/acgel.html

Books

Susan M. Lark, M.D. *Fibroid Tumors & Endometriosis Self Help Book: Solving problems of heavy bleeding, cramps, pain, infertility, and other symptoms associated with fibroid tumors and endometriosis,* (Celestial Arts, $16.95)

Asara Tsehai. *The Ancient Principles of Radiant Health: The Philosophies of an African American Woman on Health & Vitality* (510-268-1720; *www.radianthealthnow.com*)

EXERCISE

The Bodywise Woman, the Melpomene Institute staff for Women's Health, Human Kinetics (Champagne, IL) 1993.

Complete Book of Fitness Walking, James M. Rippe, Simon & Schuster, 1990.

A Hard Road to Glory: The History of the African-American Athlete, Arthur Ashe, Amistad Press, 1993.

The Joy of Walking: More Than Just Exercise, Stephen Christopher Joyner, Betterway Books (Cincinnati), 1992.

Walk for Life, David Balboa and Deena Balboa, Perigee Books, 1990.

Walk It Off!: 20 Minutes a Day to Health and Fitness, Suzanne Levine, Plume, 1991.

Victoria Johnson's Attitude: An Inspirational Guide to Redefining Your Body, Health, and Your Outlook, Victoria Johnson, Penguin Books.

SELF-ESTEEM

In the Company of My Sisters: Black Women and Self-Esteem by Julia Boyd (New York: Dutton, 1993)

HEALTHY LIVING

Black Women in America: An Historical Encyclopedia edited by Darlene Clark Hine (New York: Carlson Publishing, 1993)

Body and Soul: The Black Woman's Guide to Good Health edited by Linda Villarosa (New York: Harcourt, 1994)

Soul to Soul: A Vegetarian Soul Food Cookbook by Mary Burgess McKinney (PO Box 11476, Colton, CA 92324)

PERIODICALS

American Health
28 West 23rd Street
New York, NY 10010

Body, Mind & Spirit
255 Hope Street
Providence, RI 02906

Heart and Soul
A Health Magazine for African Americans
33 East Minor Street
Emmaus, PA 18098
215-967-8486

Natural Health
PO Box 1200
Brookline Village, MA 02147

New Age Journal
342 Wesyern Avenue
Brighton, MA 02135

Prevention
33 East Minor Street
Emmaus, PA 18098

Vegetarian Journal
The Vegetarian Resource Group
PO Box 1463
Baltimore, MD 21203

Vegetarian Times
PO Box 570
Oak Park, IL 60303

Your Health
Globe International
5401 NW Broken Sound Blvd.
Boca Raton, FL 33487

Yoga Journal
2054 University Avenue
Berkeley, CA 94704

NOTES

Chapter 1: Why Me?

1. Herbert A. Goldfarb, M.D., F.A.C.O.G., *The No-Hysterectomy Option: Your Body—Your Choice* (New York: John Wiley, 1997), 40.

2. *Comprehensive Gynecology* (Mosby), pg. 467.

3. Uterine Fibroids, http://www.womens-health.co.uk/fibroids.htm.

4. Johanna Skilling, *Fibroids: The Complete Guide to Taking Charge of Your Physical, Emotional, and Sexual Well-Being* (New York: Marlowe & Company, 2000), 5.

5. Burton Goldberg and the editors of Alternative Medicine, *Alternative Medicine Guide: Women's Health Series: Clinically Proven Alternative Therapies for Relief from Women's Health Conditions* (California: Future Medicine Publishing, 1998), 463.

6. Johanna Skilling, *Fibroids: The Complete Guide to Taking Charge of Your Physical, Emotional, and Sexual Well-Being* (New York: Marlowe & Company, 2000), 2.

7. The Fibroid Zone: http://www.womens-health.co.uk/fibroids.htm, *All About Fibroids.*

8. Women's Health: http://www.ahrq.gov/research/nov96/ra1.htm#head6: *Uterine fibroids occur more often among black women than white women undergoing hysterectomy.*

9. Ibid.

10. The Fibroid Zone: http://www.womens-health.co.uk/fibroids.htm, *All About Fibroids.*

11. Women's Health: http://www.ahrq.gov/research/nov96/ra1.htm#head6: *Uterine fibroids occur more often among black women than white women undergoing hysterectomy.*

12. Editors of Prevention Health Books, *Women's Choices in Natural Healing: Drug Free Remedies from the World of Alternative Medicine* (Emmaus, Pa.: Rodale Press, 1998), 463.

13. Obgyn.net, Theories of Fibroids, reprinted courtesy Brigham and Women's Hospital, (www.obgyn.net/ah/articles/theories_fibroids.htm).

14. Bridgette York, Fibroid News, http://freespace.virgin.net/elena/fibroidalarm.html.

15. Ziba Kashef, *Like a Natural Woman: The Black Woman's Guide to Alternative Healing* (New York: Kensington Publishing, 2001), 154.

16. Uterine Fibroids, http://www.womens-health.co.uk/fibroids.htm.

17. Health Square: http://www.healthsquare.com/fgwh/wh1ch07.htm, *Your Treatment Options for Fibroids* (From the *PDR Family Guide to Women's Health*, Chapter 7).

18. Johanna Skilling, *Fibroids: The Complete Guide to Taking Charge of Your Physical, Emotional, and Sexual Well-Being* (New York: Marlowe & Company, 2000), 108.

19. "What Every Black Woman Should Know About Fibroid Tumours," *Ebony*, March 1998, 54, 55, 59.

20. Johanna Skilling, *Fibroids: The Complete Guide to Taking Charge of Your Physical, Emotional, and Sexual Well-Being* (New York: Marlowe & Company, 2000), 16.

21. Ibid.

22. Ibid.

Chapter 2: Sizing Up Your Symptoms

1. FibroidZone, *All About Fibroids* . . . http://www.womens-health.co.uk/fibroids.htm.

2. Johanna Skilling, *Fibroids: The Complete Guide to Taking Charge of Your Physical, Emotional, and Sexual Well-Being* (New York: Marlowe & Company, 2000), 17.

3. Ibid.

4. "What Every Black Woman Should Know About Fibroid Tumours," *Ebony* March 1998, 54, 55, 59.

5. Women's Health: http://www.ahcpr.gov/research/nov96/ra1.htm.

6. Your Treatment Options for Fibroids: http://www.healthsquare.com/fgwh/wh1ch07.htm.

7. Johanna Skilling, *Fibroids: The Complete Guide to Taking Charge of Your Physical, Emotional, and Sexual Well-Being* (New York: Marlowe & Company, 2000), 21.

8. Ibid.

9. Ibid.

10. William H. Parker, M.D., with Rachel L. Parker, *A Gynecologist's Second Opinion: The Questions and Answers You Need to Take Charge of Your Health* (New York: Plume/Penguin, 1996), 22.

11. Ibid. 40.

12. FibroidZone, *All About Fibroids* . . . .http://www.womens-health.co.uk/fibroids.htm.

13. William H. Parker, M.D., with Rachel L. Parker, *A Gynecologist's Second Opinion: The Questions and Answers You Need to Take Charge of Your Health* (New York: Plume/Penguin, 1996), 28.

14. Johanna Skilling, *Fibroids: The Complete Guide to Taking Charge of Your Physical, Emotional, and Sexual Well-Being* (New York: Marlowe & Company, 2000), 184.

15. "What Every Black Woman Should Know About Fibroid Tumours," *Ebony* March 1998, 54, 55, 59. According to Nelson H. Stringer, M.D., an obstetrician/gynecologist at Rush–Presbyterian–St. Luke's Medical Center in Chicago.

Chapter 3: What's Up Doc?

1. FibroidZone, *All About Fibroids . . .* http://www.womens-health.co.uk/fibroids.htm.

2. *Black Enterprise,* August 2000.

3. Ibid.

4. GYN 101 http://www.gyn101.com/indexE.htm.

5. Ibid.

6. William H. Parker, M.D., with Rachel L. Parker, *A Gynecologist's Second Opinion: The Questions and Answers You Need to Take Charge of Your Health* (New York: Plume/Penguin, 1996), 8.

Chapter 4: Decisions, Decisions, Decisions

1. Johanna Skilling, *Fibroids: The Complete Guide to Taking Charge of Your Physical, Emotional, and Sexual Well-Being* (New York: Marlowe & Company, 2000), 50.

2. Burton Goldberg and the editors of Alternative Medicine, *Women's Health Series: Clinically Proven Alternative Therapies for Relief from Women's Health Concerns,* 103.

3. Johanna Skilling, *Fibroids: The Complete Guide to Taking Charge of Your Physical, Emotional, and Sexual Well-Being* (New York: Marlowe & Company, 2000), 52.

4. H. Winter Griffith, M.D., *Women's Health: A Guide to Symptoms, Illness, Surgery, Medical Tests and Procedures* (Berkley Publishing Group, 1999), 102.

5. Johanna Skilling, *Fibroids: The Complete Guide to Taking Charge of Your Physical, Emotional, and Sexual Well-Being* (New York: Marlowe & Company, 2000), 64.

6. Ibid., 54.

7. H. Winter Griffith, M.D., *Women's Health: A Guide to Symptoms, Illness, Surgery, Medical Tests and Procedures* (Berkley Publishing Group, 1999), 136.

8. Ibid., 57.

9. Ibid., 54.

10. FibroidZone, *All About Fibroids . . .* http://www.womens-health.co.uk/fibroids.htm

Chapter 5: Doctor's "Can Do" List

1. Carol A. Turkington with Susan J. Probst, M.D., *The Unofficial Guide to Women's Health* (IDG Books Worldwide, 2000), 131.
2. Ibid., 131.
3. William H. Parker, M.D., with Rachel L. Parker, *A Gynecologist's Second Opinion: The Questions and Answers You Need to Take Charge of Your Health* (New York: Plume/Penguin, 1996), 34.
4. Ibid., 35.
5. Ibid., 37.
6. *Essence* August 2001, "Doctors We Love: Outstanding Black OB-GYNs Take Good Care of Sisters," 74.
7. William H. Parker, M.D., with Rachel L. Parker, *A Gynecologist's Second Opinion: The Questions and Answers You Need to Take Charge of Your Health* (New York: Plume/Penguin, 1996), 43.
8. Johanna Skilling, *Fibroids: The Complete Guide to Taking Charge of Your Physical, Emotional, and Sexual Well-Being* (New York: Marlowe & Company, 2000), 92.
9. HealthLink, Agency for Health Care Quality and Research (March 1, 2000), http://healthlink.mcw.edu/article/954373368.html.
10. Ibid., 112.
11. Queen Afua, *Sacred Woman: A Guide to Healing the Feminine Body, Mind and Spirit* (Ballantine Books, 2001), 1–2.
12. Johanna Skilling, *Fibroids: The Complete Guide to Taking Charge of Your Physical, Emotional, and Sexual Well-Being* (New York: Marlowe & Company, 2000), 104.

Chapter 6: Au Naturel Remedies

1. Ziba Kashef, *Like a Natural Woman: The Black Woman's Guide to Alternative Healing* (Kensington Publishing, 2001), 72.
2. Ibid., 73.

Chapter 7: The F-Word

1. Dr. Gary Null, *The Woman's Encyclopedia of Natural Healing: The New Healing Techniques of 100 Leading Alternative Health Practitioners* (Seven Stories, 1996), 93.
2. Nelson H. Stringer, M.D., *Uterine Fibroids: What Every Woman Needs to Know* (Physicians & Scientists Publishing Co., 1996), 32.
3. Ibid., 34.
4. Dr. Gary Null, *The Woman's Encyclopedia of Natural Healing: The New Healing Techniques of 100 Leading Alternative Health Practitioners* (Seven Stories, 1996), 93.

5. Johanna Skilling, *Fibroids: The Complete Guide to Taking Charge of Your Physical, Emotional, and Sexual Well-Being* (New York: Marlowe & Company, 2000), 160.

6. Ibid., 153.

7. Susan M. Love, M.D., *Dr. Susan Love's Hormone Book: Making Informed Choices About Menopause* (New York: Three Rivers Press, 1998),

Chapter 8: Fibroid Shape-Up

1. Linda Villarosa, *Body & Soul: The Black Woman's Guide to Physical and Emotional Well-Being* (HarperPerennial, 1994), 34.

2. Michael Castleman, *Nature's Cures: From Acupressure & Aromatherapy to Walking & Yoga, the Ultimate Guide to the Best Scientifically Proven, Drug-Free Healing Methods* (New York: Bantam, 1996), 170.

Chapter 9: Techniques of Touch

1. Dr. Gary Null, *The Woman's Encyclopedia of Natural Healing: The New Healing Techniques of 100 Leading Alternative Health Practitioners* (Seven Stories, 1996), 95.

2. William Collinge, M.P.H., Ph.D., *The American Holistic Health Association Complete Guide to Alternative Medicine* (New York: Warner Books, 1997)

3. Sara Lomax Reese and Kirk Johnson with Therman Evans, M.D., *Nature's Cures: From Acupressure & Aromatherapy to Walking & Yoga, the Ultimate Guide to the Best Scientifically Proven, Drug-Free Healing Methods* (New York: Bantam, 1996), 92.

4. Mildred Carter and Tammy Carter, *Hand Reflexology: Key to Perfect Health* (Englewood Cliffs, NJ: Prentice-Hall, 2000).

Chapter 10: Heal Thyself

1. Christiane Northrup, M.D., *Women's Bodies, Women's Wisdom: Creating Physical and Emotional Healing* (Bantam, 1998), 188.

2. Sara Lomax Reese and Kirk Johnson, *HealthQuest Staying Strong: Reclaiming the Wisdom of African American Healing* (Whole Care Health, 1999), 229.

3. www.voiceofwomen.com/articles/fibroids.html.

Chapter 11: Pillow Talk

1. Johanna Skilling, *Fibroids: The Complete Guide to Taking Charge of Your Physical, Emotional, and Sexual Well-Being* (New York: Marlowe & Company, 2000), 172.

2. Ibid., 175.
3. Ibid., 178.

Chapter 12: Copycat Syndromes

1. William H. Parker, M.D., with Rachel L. Parker, *A Gynecologist's Second Opinion: The Questions and Answers You Need to Take Charge of Your Health* (New York: Plume/Penguin, 1996), 99.
2. Ibid, 243.
3. Ibid, 254.
4. Yvonne Thornton, M.D., M.P.H., *Woman to Woman: A Leading Gynecologist Tells You All You Need to Know About Your Body and Your Health* (New York: Plume, 1997), 240.
5. Ibid., 240.

Chapter 13: Oh Baby!

1. William H. Parker, M.D., with Rachel L. Parker, *A Gynecologist's Second Opinion: The Questions and Answers You Need to Take Charge of Your Health* (New York: Plume/Penguin, 1996), 28.
2. Johanna Skilling, *Fibroids: The Complete Guide to Taking Charge of Your Physical, Emotional, and Sexual Well-Being* (New York: Marlowe & Company, 2000), 182.
3. *Suburban Styles*, Fall/Winter 1998, "Infertility and You: Understanding the Causes and Seeking Treatment," 42.
4. Nelson H. Stringer, M.D., *Uterine Fibroids: What Every Woman Needs to Know* (Physicians & Scientists Publishing Co., 1996), 49.
5. Ibid., 50.
6. Johanna Skilling, *Fibroids: The Complete Guide to Taking Charge of Your Physical, Emotional, and Sexual Well-Being* (New York: Marlowe & Company, 2000), 183.
7. Herbert A. Goldfarb, M.D., F.A.C.O.G., *The No-Hysterectomy Option: Your Body, Your Choice* (New York: Wiley), 44.
8. Johanna Skilling, *Fibroids: The Complete Guide to Taking Charge of Your Physical, Emotional, and Sexual Well-Being* (New York: Marlowe & Company, 2000), 193.
9. Ibid., 197.
10. Nelson H. Stringer, M.D., *Uterine Fibroids: What Every Woman Needs to Know* (Physicians & Scientists Publishing Co., 1996), 49.

Chapter 14: No Baby!

1. Linda Villarosa, *Body & Soul: The Black Woman's Guide to Physical and Emotional Well-Being* (HarperPerennial, 1994), 164.
2. Ibid., 177.
3. Ibid., 183.

Chapter 15: Making Connections

1. Ibid., 386.
2. Ibid., 378.

INDEX